# Go Paleo?

## feeding the urban caveman

# Go Paleo?

## feeding the urban caveman

### Eve Gilmore

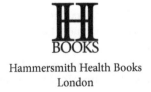

Hammersmith Health Books
London

First published in 2014 by Hammersmith Health Books – an
imprint of Hammersmith Books Limited
14 Greville Street, London EC1N 8SB, UK
www.hammersmithbooks.co.uk

British Library Cataloguing in Publication Data: A CIP record of
this book is available from the British Library.

ISBN (print edition): 978-1-78161-047-3
ISBN (ebook): 978-1-78161-048-0
Commissioning editor: Georgina Bentliff
Designed and typeset by: Julie Bennett, Bespoke Publishing Ltd
Index: Dr L Errington
Production: Helen Whitehorn, Path Projects Ltd
Printed and bound by: CPI Group (UK) Ltd, Croydon, CR0 4YY

# Contents

# Introduction

In your lifetime you are likely to eat your way through the equivalent weight of six elephants or 60,000 paperbacks. Diet has never attracted as much attention or controversy as it does today and never before has there been so much emphasis on health. In the UK we have a fitness industry telling us how to move about, a weight loss industry worth £2 billion a year, and a sickness industry known as the National Health Service, which is now bankrupt. In spite of all the resources directed towards health, in Britain today 60 per cent of adults and almost a third of children are overweight and minor health problems such as low energy compromise the ability of many of us to live life to the full.

Old age is no longer viewed as a positive final chapter distinguished by independence, wisdom and experience. Instead it has become the spectre overshadowing our middle years and looked upon with dread, if looked upon at all, as it is nearly always synonymous with degeneration or loss of dignity. So is decline an inevitable part of the ageing process and should you therefore accept your fate with equanimity, or could it be that you have the power to shape your health destiny?

It appears that rather than being deterministic, genes are turned on and off by environmental triggers including diet. This puts us firmly behind the wheel and shifts our genes into the back seat from where they may proffer helpful navigational advice, but whether we take it is up to each of us. Freeing yourself from the media bandwagon, which tends to lurch from one health fad to another, and learning how to thrive rather than survive could be the most life-changing decision you will ever make – for you *and* your family. You won't, however, learn how to do this by looking at the tip of the disease iceberg, as disease strikes when the system becomes overloaded and the body-boat is starting to sink. Expelling unwanted cargo, steering towards calmer seas and getting the boat ship-shape again are better options than simply plugging the symptom holes.

In *Go Paleo?* you will discover how the modern diet increases your risk of chronic disease and why a way of eating based on hunter-gatherer or 'Paleo' *principles* is one of the most effective means of offloading unnecessary cargo and setting your ship towards calmer waters. If you would like to know what to feed your family, or can answer 'yes' to any of the following questions, this book might be just what you have been waiting for:

- I don't have as much energy as I used to
- I have niggling problems, like allergies, headaches or indigestion
- I have irritable bowel or sometimes feel bloated
- I would like to sleep better
- My concentration and memory are poor
- I sometimes feel depressed for no reason
- I am less able to cope with stress and sometimes feel over-anxious
- I get irritable if I am hungry
- I would like to lose weight but have difficulty controlling what I eat or cannot lose weight in spite of eating less
- I feel stiff and achy first thing
- I have hormonal or fertility problems.

Good health and vitality are your birth right, so let's widen our perspective and go far back to a time when disease was unknown. The evolutionary model can tell us everything we need to know about the lifestyle best suited to our caveman genes – which have hardly changed in millennia. Our Stone Age ancestors, and the few remaining hunter-gatherers, are noted for their stamina, athletic physique and *absence of disease*. This wasn't because they led short, brutal lives. Provided they survived infancy they could expect to enjoy a long and healthy lifespan. The sad truth is today, from pasty-faced couch potatoes to those sweating it out in the gym, we are poor specimens in comparison. Virtually non-existent before the Industrial Revolution, digestive problems have become widespread amongst all age groups and it is estimated that between 60 and 70 million people worldwide suffer from indigestion or poor bowel function. Puberty often marks the onset of hormonal problems, acne or mental health disorders; and infertility is rising exponentially amongst those of child-bearing age. Cardiovascular disease and diabetes, formerly only affecting the elderly, are striking at a younger age, whilst chronic diseases generally continue to rise.

Today it is sometimes said that we are digging our graves with our knife and fork. Food and agriculture have become big business and when money is involved facts tend to get lost. Science has been hi-jacked by those who can pay the highest prices, and in the mainstream media 'news' relating to health may actually be little more than marketing copy. This is one of the reasons why there is so much conflicting advice about health and diet. Millions are spent on generating misinformation purporting to be about health but which is often promoting foods produced by the industry itself or dissuading people from eating foods which are less profitable to produce. Healthy profits tend to come before healthy people. Furthermore, research is expensive and undertaking it has become inaccessible to all but the highest bidders, making it almost impossible to obtain unbiased information. Meanwhile, the juggernaut of health dogma that has infiltrated medical thinking, the food industry and the media ploughs on. Within a few decades foods previously considered healthy, such as animal fats and red meat, have been demonised, even though they have been the mainstay of the human diet for millions of years.

So instead of throwing money at disease in an attempt to understand how to suppress it, it can be more revealing to study what promotes health. The evolutionary model suggests that the Paleo diet, low in carbohydrate and high in saturated fats and animal produce, may represent the optimal way of eating. Enjoyed by humans for over two and a half million years, study after study has associated the hunter-gatherer diet with strength, longevity and the absence of disease.

## So what is the Paleo diet?

First, it is important to state there is no such thing as 'the Paleo diet' per se. Pre-agricultural diets were regionally variable and seasonally cyclical. In colder climates they tended to be meat-based as the land was either under snow for much of the year or of poor quality and only suited to grazing. In warmer regions fewer red meats were eaten and fruits and plants dominated. Although the ancestral diet may have varied in content, it was more nutrient dense than that of today. So although no standardised Paleo diet exists, the Paleo diet is usually defined by what it excludes, and is generally accepted as being grain, legume and dairy free.

It is thought that the advent of agriculture around 10,000 years ago marked the demise of the nomadic way of life, giving way to the cultivation of grains and legumes and the domestication of animals for milk. Archaeological remains suggest an abrupt decline in health at this time. Loss of stature, arthritis and other diseases associated with poor mineralisation seem to coincide with the introduction of grains into the diet. Ten thousand years might seem like a long time to those of us who hope to live to around 80 but is, in fact, the evolutionary equivalent of the 'blink of an eye', and would not have given us enough time to adapt. However, there is archaeological evidence that some hunter-gatherers were eating grains much earlier than this. It seems the closer to the equator, the greater the intake of plant-based foods, which in some cases may have included wild grains. This may explain why gluten (and dairy) intolerance is more prevalent in colder latitudes, and why those with Scandinavian or north European ancestry are poorly suited to a vegetarian diet. What the hunter gatherer diets seemed to have in common was that they were highly nutritious and all contained meat or fish. They provided good levels of minerals, saturated fat and fat soluble vitamins, with little or no grain or dairy and variable amounts of protein, most of which was derived from meat. Much of the diet was raw which further increased the nutrient density and provided good levels of fibre. I suspect that rather than being historically accurate, the modern assumption that the Paleo diet was a high protein diet results from the misplaced fat and carb phobia that is still influencing nutritional thinking today. In fact, the food group most highly prized in the ancestral diet was saturated fat. Carbs have been given a bad press because they are nearly always derived from grains, a food group that causes problems in a number of people. However, carbs from vegetables and fruits are much easier for the body to handle. A diet high in raw vegetables and salads does not have the same effect as a diet high in cereals, although both are high in carbohydrate. Whilst it may seem impossible to imagine a diet without grains, they are easily replaced by alternatives such as vegetable pastas, and coconut, seed and nut flours in baking and bread making. Nuts can be fermented into cheeses, coconut cream into yoghurt and soft cheese, and the milk from nuts and coconuts can be made into delicious desserts and ice-creams, making Paleo eating varied and enjoyable.

What is also known about the Paleo diet is that it contained virtually no sugar. Refining has enabled us to concentrate sugars in quantities that our bodies are ill equipped to handle. For example, a soft drink contains the equivalent of eight and a half feet of sugar cane – an impossible quantity to get through in its unrefined state. The high proportion of carbohydrates in the modern diet compounds our inbuilt predilection for sweet foods. Until technology got involved in food production, foods that were bitter were generally poisonous and those that were sweet were usually safe to eat, but that doesn't apply today since many foods are laced with sugar, high-fructose corn syrup and artificial sweeteners – and they definitely aren't safe to eat. Our first food, breast milk, contains a sugar called lactose and thus the early association between feeding and being loved is established before we are capable of conscious thought. Eating is associated with emotion, and this is one of the reasons sweet foods can be comforting, and why we can feel deprived and miserable when trying to give them up.

Despite their pervasive presence at nearly every meal today, in Europe and America grains were only elevated from animal fodder to dietary staple at the time of the Industrial Revolution, cultivating in us a taste for stodgy, high-carbohydrate foods, which has been a contributory factor to the obesity epidemic. The Arabic nations seem to have been eating grains the longest, and there wheat sensitivity and carbohydrate intolerance are rare. The rapid increase in degenerative disease that has characterised the last 100 years demonstrates that most of us have struggled to adapt. It is estimated that 80 per cent of cancers are related in some way to diet, and it is probably evident to you that much of the food we eat today could not be described as healthy.

In fact, much of it wouldn't be recognised by even our recent ancestors. Not only are the foods themselves different – the result of selective cultivation or the products of technology – but the ratios of fat, protein and carbohydrate have been reversed. Fat phobia flourishes, and grains – previously dismissed as mostly animal feed, as I have said – now form the foundation of almost everything we eat. In addition, some of what passes for food isn't food at all but a concoction of chemicals, conceived in the laboratory rather than grown on the land. Modern grass eaters, particularly cows, may not have had access to grass, and non-organic crops will have been forced to grow in demineralised soils, which is why today's produce contains an average of 80 per cent less nutrients than it did only 50 years ago.

## Are we getting healthier?

It is a common misconception that we have never been healthier and enjoy greater longevity due to advances in modern medicine. We are most definitely healthier than our under-nourished and over-worked predecessors who lived in squalor whilst servicing the factories and mills of the Industrial Revolution – a time when health hit an all-time low – but we are not anything like as healthy as our hunter-gatherer ancestors. Today, the cost of healthcare is escalating, but people are getting sicker. The expense of caring for the increasingly decrepit ageing population is eating into inheritances, and degenerative disease, which has increased by nearly 400 per cent in a century, is striking at a younger age. The emergence of special needs schools and the increase in obesity in children are further evidence of the declining state of health in the civilised world.

Statistics serve to confound as they indicate that, on average, we are living longer than our recent ancestors. However, once infant mortality rates and deaths from wars, epidemics, accidents and childbirth are removed, those who survived such early challenges would have been expected to have lived well into old age, and without the degenerative diseases that afflict us today. Contrary to popular belief, advances in medicine have had no impact whatsoever on our lifespan[1] – quite the reverse – and our health has actually deteriorated exponentially alongside so-called advances in medicine. The United States of America, which spends more than any other country on health and is the most medicated society in the world, is the sickest on the planet – and also the fattest.

The last 100 years have seen dramatic shifts in causes of death that correlate with the rapid changes in our diets and lifestyles. In 1900 acute diseases or accidents accounted for 70 per cent of all deaths, with degenerative (chronic) diseases being responsible for the other 30 per cent. Today the situation has reversed, with chronic diseases accounting for more than 70 per cent of all mortalities. So commonplace are diseases in the elderly they are considered to be age-related – the inevitable result of the body wearing out rather than the accumulative effects of decades of eating the wrong diet and living in a polluted environment.

That is not to suggest that in the past everyone enjoyed robust health and was free from disease, because that was most certainly not the case. Poverty has always negatively affected health, not only through impaired nutrition but also because of harsh living and working conditions. The point is that modern health problems, such as cardiovascular disease and diabetes, were almost unknown until relatively recently. So rare were heart attacks in the early 20th century that most doctors would never have encountered one throughout their entire professional career.

Today, 7 per cent of Americans are diagnosed with cardiovascular disease, making it the most common cause of death in the Western world.

In the past, infectious diseases tended to predominate, and the plague regularly decimated populations across Europe and beyond. Changes in lifestyle factors, including diet, have resulted in a dramatic shift in disease demographics over the last century, with the last 30 decades witnessing declining health in the young. There is an exponential increase in mental illness, behavioural and learning problems and allergies in children, and degenerative disease striking before middle age. The sudden change from acute, infectious diseases to chronic in less than 100 years cannot be explained away by 'genetics', since our genes have hardly changed in over 2 million years.

## The Industrial Revolution – a revolution in health

Flora Thompson wrote the book *Larkrise to Candleford* at the onset of the Industrial Revolution but it is set some 30 years earlier. An account of a way of life that was fast disappearing, Thompson describes how people used to enjoy long, healthy lives working on the land until old age, when they succumbed to rheumatism as a result of living and working in cold, damp conditions. They seldom had need of doctors, barring accidents. The local midwife would attend at childbirth, and most women had a working knowledge of herbal remedies which they used to treat common ailments. Allergies, mental illness, obesity and many of the other problems that afflict us today were unknown. People ate fresh, seasonal produce, drank unpasteurised milk, baked sourdough breads, and cured their own bacon from a fatted pig which saw them through the winter. It was only when the population was suddenly uprooted from the country, and transported into overcrowded and unhygienic conditions to service the mills and factories that sprang up during that time that disease set in.

The Industrial Revolution represented a dramatic change in lifestyle, living conditions and nutrition. Fresh produce became a distant memory whilst refined and processed foods became staples of the new diet. Since that time, the biggest positive impact on health has been due to improved hygiene and sanitation, which has reduced the spread of infectious disease. *It has not been due to the development of pharmaceutical drugs.*

Prior to the Industrial Revolution, most of our ancestors eked out a rural existence from the land. Out in all weathers, they were used to hard manual labour. This applied to women as well as men, who coped with domestic chores without the labour-saving devices of today, a feat that would have been impossible had they suffered from modern complaints like low energy and bad backs, for example. Indeed, anthropological and historical evidence suggests that they were far more robust than we are. Leaving aside the rise in infectious diseases linked to urban over-crowding, dangerous working conditions and lack of sanitation, stamina and strength declined rapidly during the Industrial Revolution. This was the first time in history that people lived many miles away from where their food was produced, and new methods of production, preservation and transportation had to be developed. It was realised that refining could extend the shelf life of flour – probably because the weevil was more discerning than man – and thus refined flour, with 80 per cent of its nutrients removed, was first foisted on an unsuspecting population.

Traditional methods of salting and curing meats gave way to canning, and preservatives were added to foods in the form of chemicals. In fact, so well preserved are we today that it now takes longer for our bodies to decompose after death – unless we're cremated in which case we release a noxious vapour laden with heavy metals and chemicals into the surrounding atmosphere.

For the first time ever, food production was removed from the population who ate it, becoming centrally produced and then transported by the newly invented steam trains and boats. The diet shifted overnight from seasonal farm-fare of fresh meats, vegetables and fruit to a more grain-based diet, and it was not until the later invention of refrigeration that fresh produce became widely available again. Until then, urban dwellers had to eat preserved meats, pickled or canned fruits and vegetables, and baked goods. Consequently, there was a substantial decrease in the nutritional content of the food and this, in combination with the squalor in which they lived, proved disastrous for many as infectious diseases and malnutrition took hold.

The removal of the population from food production is significant and heralded many changes in what was eaten and how. Plant foods start to lose nutrients as soon as they have been picked, but for the working classes, fresh food had become a thing of the past. All of this constituted a revolutionary and rapid change in diet to which we have been unable to adapt, and from which we are still reeling today. Digestive problems and obesity first started to manifest around 1800 and have continued to increase ever since. Autoimmune diseases such as rheumatoid arthritis began to appear for the first time, and deficiency diseases started to affect rural and urban populations alike. Problems included reduced stature, postural weakness (bad backs), dental caries (tooth decay), arthritis, and diabetes, the legacy of which looms large today.

Obviously, modern lifestyle factors are also relevant and some of these are examined in my other books. It is, however, indisputable that a good diet is fundamental to health. What constitutes a good diet continues to be the subject of much debate, although it is generally accepted that refined foods, chemical additives and sugar are not good for us. Furthermore, since grains are high in carbohydrate, and carbohydrate is converted to sugar in the body, it is not difficult to surmise that increased grain and sugar consumption are almost certainly contributing to our health problems.

Studies on modern hunter-gatherers – who only suffer from degenerative diseases upon switching to the 'civilised' diet – have revealed that indigenous eating seems to confer a protective effect. However, their numbers are dwindling as the Western way of life encroaches on the natural world like waves bringing in the tide. Researchers now tend to focus on the disease itself rather than on the person who has the disease, or the environment within which that person lives. Lifespans and memories are short, and it takes only one generation for something new to become the norm. Autism, behavioural problems and asthma in children illustrate this point well. Rare 30 years ago, schools now have to employ assistants to chaperone their more challenging pupils. Asthma pumps have proliferated in the medical cupboards like mushrooms on a wet night, and are now used by around one third of children.

Furthermore, lifestyle factors which are now exerting a multi-generational effect can make it difficult to attribute one aspect – in this case diet – to changes in health. For example, hunter-gatherers are more active and less exposed to environmental pollution than we are, and the reality is that most diseases are multi-factorial. Our lives have changed so much over the last hundred years that in order to fully understand the ways in which the modern world affects our health, we have to take a broader view and employ a little common sense.

We have to free ourselves from our love affair with the double-blind-placebo-controlled trial, which can obfuscate the blindingly obvious. Hiding behind 'the need for more research' the industry employs the so-called scientific method to delay the release of incriminating evidence until it becomes irrefutable. It doesn't require a scientific background, and indeed may even be advantageous not to have one, to work out that living in a toxic environment whilst eating a diet of industrially produced, poor quality foods is unlikely to be conducive to health. Like smoking, the picture is blurred by the smokescreen of 'lack of scientific proof', which actually means the industry will get away with it until the evidence becomes irrefutable and the 'scientists' on the corporate payroll are unable to stem the backlash. Unfortunately, since the effects of a poor diet, or toxic exposure, can take decades to manifest, time appears to favour the industry. Rather than erring on the side of caution, and despite mounting environmental damage, toxic and polluting practices are always assumed to be safe.

In dispelling many modern dietary myths, *Go Paleo?* examines what is currently understood about diet and health and invites you to decide how and what you want to eat, although this may change according to your age, health and circumstances. There is probably no single food that would be good for everyone. Your first loyalty is to your body and not to a philosophy no matter how grandiose and persuasive it may be. Buffered against the vagaries of changing health advice and fad diets designed to trick rather than nourish the body, *Go Paleo?* explains why the modern diet puts the body under stress and is nutritionally inferior to Stone Age diets. To what extent these diets could be replicated today is unclear. Whether it would be practical or even desirable is doubtful. What is certain is that the modern diet is made up of denatured foods at odds with our genetic blueprint.

To get some idea of how differently we eat today consider how empty your local supermarket would be if it were stripped of anything unavailable in Paleo times. Gone would be the cereals, ready-meals, breads, pasteurised dairy produce, tinned beans, biscuits, cakes, confectionery, soft drinks, etc. Gone too would be most fruits and vegetables as selective breeding has made them completely different from their wild counterparts. For instance, the nightshade family (potatoes, tomatoes, peppers and aubergines) was poisonous, wild carrot contained natural pesticides making it bitter and inedible, and the presence of cyanide would have put almonds and apricots off the menu. Most vegetables familiar to us today did not exist, and bone marrow, organs and glands were preferred. Intensively reared, low-fat muscle meat and farmed or contaminated fish bear no resemblance nutritionally to the wild meats enjoyed by our ancestors.

Humans appear to be omnivorous, which means they are neither vegetarian nor carnivorous but can eat a varied diet of plant and animal foods. We can learn much from anthropological studies, and even though we cannot replicate the ancestral diet today, we can improve our health by applying some of the principles. The best source of information about 20th-century hunter-gatherer diets was compiled by Dr Weston A Price who studied a total of 14 indigenous cultures and recorded his findings in the seminal book *Nutrition and Physical Degeneration*.

Criticism of Paleo eating is almost always directed at the modern version of the diet, which is generally high in lean protein and low in salt and fat, even though there is no anthropological evidence to support this. This is Stone Age eating seen through the prism of modern health dogma. Dr Price found traditional diets to consist of up to 65 per cent fat, most of which was saturated, with a protein intake of between 10 and 20 per cent. The high-protein hybrid of Stone Age eating currently gaining popularity amongst the fitness industry is not, in my view, representative of Paleo eating. The explorer and anthropologist Vilhjalmur Stefansson, who lived amongst the Inuit and Native Americans at the beginning of the 20th century, observed that lean meat was avoided. Protein without fat is toxic and Stefansson himself succumbed to ill health when his doctors put him on a low-fat, lean-meat diet – a diet that was quickly revoked once they saw its effects.

I have been recommending my version of Paleo eating called *The Urban Caveman diet* since 2006. It is a diet adapted to modern tastes and based on what I understand the principles of Stone Age eating to be. We have to take into account the foods available, and the environment and lifestyle that inform the bodies we now inhabit. We cannot pretend we are hunter-gatherers foraging for wild foods. When asked for directions, the apocryphal Irishman replied, 'I wouldn't start from here,' but we have to start from here. Not everyone can move from junk food to health food in one easy leap. Some non-Paleo foods are important for restoring health and some health problems respond better to non-Paleo diets.

Over the years, I have tried almost every diet under the sun – both professionally and personally. From vegetarianism and veganism in the '80s to low-fat, high-fat, low-carb, high-carb, no-carb after 6 pm, low-protein, high-protein, raw food, anti-Candida, food combining – sadly the list goes on. My ah-ha moment came in 2006 when I attended a conference on autoimmune disease presented by one of Dr Loren Cordain's team at Colorado University, which is the centre for research into Paleo eating. Imagine my excitement at the prospect of yet another diet! Out went the grain and dairy and I was eating what I *thought* to be Paleo within hours of having left the conference.

Having noticed immediate benefits myself, it wasn't long before many of my clients were eating this way too. It soon dawned on me that what most diets have in common is that they are attempts at minimising the effects of the modern diet on the body. Barely a year goes by without a new miracle diet hitting the media. Even though previous diets promised much and delivered little, hope triumphs over experience. The need to find a better way of eating ensures a ready market for anyone claiming to have 'the answer' to our health or weight problems. Experience has taught me that nearly everyone notices improvements when cutting out grains, dairy and sugar and that their reintroduction tends to herald a downturn in energy or the return of old symptoms. This begs the question whether it is the foods themselves that are the problem, or could it be the way they have been adulterated by modern production methods? If the latter, is it even necessary to eliminate them altogether?

The biggest problem with the modern Paleo diet is the lack of familiar foods. Reared on high-carb comfort foods it is not surprising that the most common internet search for Paleo-related information is for Paleo pasta. Convenience is also important. Packed lunches become more challenging without bread for sandwiches. A strict Paleo diet actually feels like a healthy diet and this can be great for a few weeks – especially if it comes hot on the heels of over-indulgence – but after the novelty wears off and you become fed up with being virtuous, reasons for indulging in non-Paleo foods can start to become very compelling. A slice of bread here and a bar of chocolate there, and before you realise, you've slipped from a virtuous to a vicious cycle. For a diet to be a sustainable lifestyle choice it has to satisfy your gastronomic, emotional, practical and social needs. It has to become a way of life rather than a temporary gesture of self-denial or deprivation.

The great news is that it is not necessary to replicate the Paleo diet in order to improve your health. The Paleo diet needed to be adapted for the 21st-century palate as well as being visually appealing and satisfying to your inner child. Although gourmet caveman-eating hasn't yet reached the restaurant industry – and this is something I would dearly love to change – it can hold its own at any self-respecting dinner party. I hope my Urban Caveman diet successfully bridges the gap between the sensory gratification of the modern diet and the benefits of healthy eating. It is not prescriptive and gives you a range of options for substituting healthier alternatives for modern ingredients. It is for anyone who loves food and values health. You can find out more about Urban Caveman eating from www.21stcenturypaleo.com and from *The Urban Caveman Recipe Collection* which contains over 300 mouth-watering recipes. Healthy eating has never been easier or more enjoyable.

# Chapter 1

# The urban caveman

In this chapter we are going to look at what makes the Urban Caveman diet the smart choice if you want to improve your health and increase your energy. This diet offers you Paleo-friendly alternatives to common ingredients, giving you the chance to draw your own line in the sand. If, like me, you have fallen victim to diets in the past that subsequently turned out to have been little more than a health craze you will also want to be sure that you are not embarking upon yet another fad diet. Publicised almost as soon as they are formulated, dietary fads tend to spread like wildfire amongst the overweight and the eternally optimistic, often despite having little medical validation. You always start a new diet full of hope and resolve, so it can be a bitter blow if the promised results fail to materialise. It takes determination, or perhaps desperation, not to become disheartened, and if this has happened to you in the past, it is to your great credit that you are ready to stomach (pun intended) another book about diet.

How can you be sure that any new diet is going to be worthwhile? Would over 2.5 million years of historical and scientific evidence be enough to reassure you? We have been hunter-gatherers for over 2.5 million years, living off the land for most of recorded history. Over the last 500 generations grains, dairy, sugar and beans were eaten sparingly, if at all, by most hunter-gatherers and our digestive systems are not designed to process them in the quantities or form they are consumed today. In a comparatively short space of time they have come to dominate our diet whilst fat has been demoted and discredited. Furthermore, modern agricultural and production methods have so transformed the foods themselves that they can challenge even the most robust of digestive systems. Wheat and dairy have been especially affected. They are mass produced, selectively bred and subjected to treatments that turn them from food to foe for many people. This is why grains and dairy are often associated with allergies, digestive problems and autoimmune diseases and why most people feel better when avoiding them. For some, a period of elimination followed by a gradual introduction of traditionally grown and prepared grains and raw milks, enables them to be reintroduced without any problem whilst for others, a life-time of avoidance may be necessary.

In contrast, 19th- and early 20th-century researchers studying the dwindling numbers of hunter-gatherers around the planet, found them (at the time of the study) to be healthy, fit, lean and muscular. Totally absent were the diseases of 'civilisation': their blood pressure was average, there was no cancer, arthritis or heart disease, and mental health problems were unknown. Since our genes and digestive systems haven't changed since our nomadic days, it is reasonable to assume that the pre-industrial or even Paleo diet suits us better.

Dr Weston A Price, the Harvard-trained dentist and anthropologist previously mentioned, was interested in the teeth of nomads, and he travelled extensively during the 1920s and 30s, studying a total of 14 different hunter-gatherer tribes. His findings resulted in the seminal book *Nutrition and Physical Degeneration*, in which he provided photographic and medical evidence showing the impact on health of the introduction of the 'civilised diet' within one generation. This is worrying considering the relatively unadulterated diet of the first half of the 20th century. And he was not alone. Included in the book is a quote from the writings of Ernest Thompson Seton (1860–1946), who compared white settlers to the American Indians: 'The civilization of the white man is a failure; it is visibly crumbling around us.' '…All historians, hostile and friendly, admit the Indian to have been the finest type of physical manhood the world has ever known. None but the best, the picked, chosen and trained of the Whites, had any chance with him.'

Surgery has arisen from the need to remove or repair diseased organs and examination of the organs of those on the typical Western diet has shown them to be misshapen and pale. Sir Arbuthnot Lane (1856–1943), an expert on the differences between the digestive systems of modern man compared to primitives, observed: 'Long surgical experience has proved to me conclusively that there is something radically and fundamentally wrong with the civilized mode of life, and I believe that unless the present dietetic and health customs of the White Nations are reorganised, social decay and race deterioration are inevitable.'

That the above observations were made almost a century ago makes them even more alarming. Of particular relevance today is the marked decline in mental health. There is an increasing incidence of anxiety disorders, schizophrenia and depression while many others require help in managing their lives, as the numbers of children now classified as having 'special needs' testifies. The sociologist John Laird wrote in 1935: 'The country's average level of general ability sinks lower with each generation.'

This was written before the advent of intensive farming practices, and the introduction of food additives, pesticides, junk foods, high-fructose corn syrup, genetic modification and other ills associated with modern food production, and it predates autism, which was first defined by Kanner in 1943. The short attention spans of a generation reared in front of television and computer screens rather than typeface and paper have further contributed to the dumbing-down process.

Archaeological examination of the remains of our primitive

ancestors has revealed a sudden decline in health upon the introduction of grains into the diet, including loss of height by an average of six inches or 15 centimetres, an increase in infectious diseases and infant mortality, and a reduction in lifespan. Bone mineral disorders, such as rickets, osteomalacia and osteoporosis began to appear for the first time, and deficiency diseases became widespread. Teeth became rotten and overcrowded. This is because grains contain a substance called 'phytic acid' that interferes with the uptake of minerals and you can read more about this in chapter 2. Things deteriorated still further with the introduction of dairy produce and the preservation of meat.

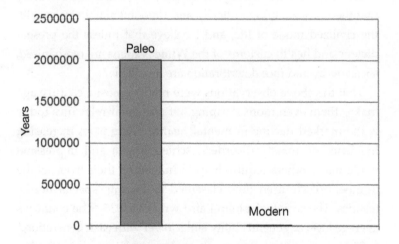

**Figure 1:** Graph showing the relatively short time we have been eating grains, dairy and legumes ('Modern') compared with eating a 'Paleo' diet.

As I have said, Weston Price studied a total of 14 different cultures that included the Australian Aboriginals, Africans, Polynesians and South Americans, all of whom were consuming the indigenous diets of their forebears. His conclusions were confirmed by the observations of other researchers, including Dr

Pottenger, who looked at the effects of different diets on cats, the explorer Stefansson, who studied and lived with the Inuit, and Dr Albert Schweitzer who visited Africa and wrote: 'I was astonished to encounter no cases of cancer… This absence of cancer seemed to be due to the difference in nutrition of the natives compared to Europeans.'

Like Sir Arbuthnot Lane previously, Pottenger also noted the poor condition of the internal organs of individuals consuming a Western diet. He fed four generations of cats on four different diets, after which he dissected them and photographed their organs. He found a difference between the healthy organs of the raw meat-fed cats compared with the bloated and discoloured organs of those fed a more processed diet. He also noticed that only the pens that had housed the cats eating the raw meat diet were able to support the growth of weeds. The other pens were barren.

Over a ten-year period, Dr Pottenger bred four generations of cats which he divided into groups according to what they were fed. The group reared on a diet of raw meat and milk remained healthy and fertile. However, the first generation of cats fed pasteurised, evaporated or condensed milk developed diseases towards the end of their lives. The second generation developed diseases in midlife, whilst the third developed diseases early in life, with many dying before six months of age. No fourth generation was produced in the latter group due to either infertility or miscarriage.

Explorer and anthropologist Stefansson (see page xxi) wrote, in *Cancer: Disease of Civilisation*, of a whaling ship's doctor who found only a single cancer case in 49 years among the Inuit of Alaska and Canada. Stefansson was a pioneer of Stone Age nutrition, living with and adopting the lifestyle and diet of the Eskimos. Whilst contemporary explorers were dependent upon tons of stored food for their expeditions, Stefansson relied only upon the animals he caught and the knowledge he had gained from the Inuit. He stopped eating vegetables and ate only meat, and at a time when Dr Kellogg was gaining popularity for his cereals this was considered impossible. Doctors at a New York Hospital studied Stefansson (and a colleague who enjoyed the same diet) over a one-year period and were amazed to discover that they thrived on it. Stefansson remained on this diet until he was 60, when he married and was enticed by his much younger wife into baked foods and deserts. Eleven years later he suffered a stroke, after which he reverted back to his Stone Age diet and made an almost complete recovery. It was during this period that he wrote his seminal book.

Weston Price, who is sometimes called the Charles Darwin of Nutrition, discovered that only when 'civilised' diets were adopted did dental caries and over-crowding of teeth appear. Hunter-gatherers had no need of dentists. The teeth are the visible part of the skeleton, and the fact that grains not only provide little in the way of minerals and that they can impede the uptake of minerals is the reason for reduced bone mineralisation, reduced stature and generalised weakness which is considered normal today. Indeed, osteoporosis is attributed to 'wear and tear' rather than decades of inadequate mineralisation of the bones and joints linked in part to a lack of saturated fat and vitamins D and K..

Back problems are said to affect 80 per cent of Americans at some time in their lives. This means that our backs are too weak to hold most of us up properly, straining the muscles and causing poor postural habits which simply perpetrate the problem. Esther Gokhale, in her book *Eight Steps to a Pain Free Back*, notes that modern hunter-gatherers when studied had excellent posture and were free of back problems.

Weston Price observed that, providing the natives reverted back to their natural diets, the next generation had straight teeth and recovered their physical prowess. More than 80 years ago he concluded: 'No era in the long journey of mankind reveals in the skeletal remains such a terrible degeneration of teeth and bones as this brief modern period records.'

## Supersize nutrition

It would be impossible to replicate the hunter-gatherer diet accurately today. For a start, the foods were wild and 100 per cent organic. Now even organically produced food is often contaminated due to the infiltration of chemicals into the natural environment. Foods can also be legally classified as organic if they have been sprayed by a pesticide called rotenone or treated with antibiotics.* There has been a campaign in the US calling for a ban on the spraying of organic apples and pears with antibiotics which is set to become law in October 2014. Organic chickens have also been found to contain antibiotics. In Britain the Soil Association defines organic as 'not routinely given antibiotics'. 'Routinely' is the industry's get-out-of-jail card and permits the use of antibiotics if there is risk of infection at the farm. Furthermore, genetic intervention and selective breeding have changed the constituents of modern foods. For example, today's fruits are much higher in fructose (sugar) than they were a few decades ago. Bananas can no longer reproduce in the wild as they no longer have seeds. Wild lettuce was too tough to digest and was not part of the ancestral diet. Today's meat comes from farmed rather than wild animals and may also have been intensively reared. For all these reasons and more, it is only possible to follow the spirit of the Paleo diet – but even that could have a positive effect on health and well-being.

Weston Price found the so-called 'primitive' diets contained at least four times the water-soluble vitamins, calcium and other minerals, and at least ten times the fat-soluble vitamins which came from animal foods, such as butter, fish and meats. 'Primitive'

---

*According to the Soil Association a 'handful of permissions (to use rotenone) are granted each year. Rotenone may be replaced by a natural pesticide called Spinosid.

cultures also appreciated the importance of pre-conceptual nutrition, placing both prospective parents on special dietary and fitness programmes to ensure the best possible health for the next generation. The foods they were given all contained high levels of animal fats, which are rich in vitamins A, D and K. It is unusual today for parents to consider pre-conceptual health and we are still encouraged to follow a low- rather than high-fat diet.

Before the advent of modern agriculture our diet consisted mostly of wild organ meats, fish, foraged eggs, vegetables, fruits, and a few nuts and seeds. Protein came from pasture-fed animals and wild fish, both of which are high in saturated fats – the fats that a few decades ago were suddenly declared unhealthy by the health police. Today, many animals that would naturally graze on grass are instead fed grains, which changes the structure and constituents of the meat and this is why meat 'allergies' have started to appear.

Since fat is needed to make energy, the recent switch to a high carb low-fat diet has spawned some of the fatigue and weight problems common today. It is obvious that were animal fats and red meat detrimental to health we would not have thrived on them for millions of years. In fact, the recent epidemic of degenerative disease has paralleled a *reduction* in the intake of meat and animal fat. Convincing the public that healthy foods like red meat and saturated fat are bad has been a marketing triumph but a health disaster. This is examined in detail in the book *Trick and Treat* by Barry Groves.

The food pyramid, that mainstay of modern dietary dogma beloved of dieticians and doctors, advocates that the bulk of the diet should be carbohydrate-based. The emphasis is therefore on bread, cereals, rice and pasta, followed by other high-carb foods, such as fruits and vegetables, with meats and fats making up only a small proportion of the diet. In reality, this pyramid needs to be turned on its head, literally and metaphorically as it represents a complete reversal of the diets enjoyed by the more slender and

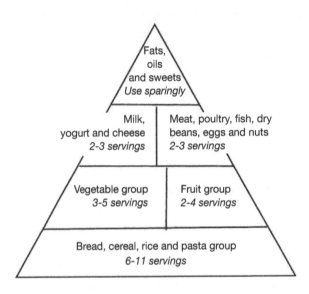

**Figure 2:** The Food Pyramid – current UK Government recommendations for the relative balance of the food groups

athletic hunter-gatherer. So, having looked at some of the evidence that supports the Paleo way of eating, we are now going to turn our attention to what it is about some of our most commonly eaten foods that makes them so difficult for us to digest.

## The Stone Age digestive system and the modern diet

Since our genes and digestive systems haven't changed since our nomadic days it is reasonable to assume that we may be better suited to the hunter-gatherer way of eating, and there is much evidence to support this view.

Humans belong to the primate family[1] and, in common with more than 95 per cent of primates, have a single-chambered stomach that is incapable of digesting most complex carbohydrates, such as grains. In contrast, herbivores have two stomachs, which enable them to digest carbohydrates in two stages, whilst granivores, such as chickens, have three pancreatic ducts that supply special enzymes to break down starches.

The human gut is different from that of most other primates as the bowel is much shorter, leaving a reduced surface area for absorbing nutrients from leaves and stems, which makes us reliant upon nutritionally dense foods, such as meat. Shorter intestines are found only in carnivores and primates that eat a largely meat-based diet. This characteristic is also linked to manual dexterity, and primates who rely upon a vegetarian diet do not possess the opposable thumb as we do.

The human pancreas is both an endocrine (hormonal) gland and a digestive organ. It produces juices and enzymes that assist in digestion in a part of the small intestine called the duodenum. Therefore, digestive functions constitute the bulk of its work, although due to the prevalence of diabetes today it is more commonly associated in most people's minds with the production of insulin. It may therefore surprise you to learn that less than 1 per cent of pancreatic cells produce insulin. This fact alone shows we do not have the capacity to cope with a predominantly carbohydrate-based diet.

A craving for sweet food after a meal can sometimes be due to the outpouring of insulin in response to excessive carbohydrate intake, only to abate when enough carbohydrate has been consumed to match the level of insulin. If you are in any doubt about grains being high in starch, look at the residue that remains in the sink after draining a saucepan of pasta. Eating a high-carb diet places a strain on the digestive system as a whole, suppresses the production of stomach acid and overloads the intestines and pancreas – not least because of the increased need for starch-splitting enzymes and the rapid spike in blood sugar which follows carb consumption.

Unfortunately, grains and legumes (peas, beans, lentils etc) create a double-whammy because they contain enzyme inhibitors to protect them against predators. These enzyme inhibitors do just what their name implies, which is to prevent starch-splitting enzymes from working, rendering the food almost indigestible, as many who suffer from embarrassing wind problems have discovered.

The cumulative effects of munching your way through mountains of carbs over many years can ultimately result in the development of **insulin resistance** or type 2 diabetes and can lay the foundations for obesity and other degenerative diseases. Over time, a grain-based diet depletes enzyme levels, resulting in fatigue and sluggish digestion, and this is partly why their avoidance nearly always produces an improvement in energy and digestion and loss of weight.

## What is the evidence that we are meant to eat Paleo?

The earliest human remains have been found on the African savannah. The savannah differs from the environment of many other primates who eat more vegetation in their diets. Herbivores live off the grasses of the savannah, and omnivores (humans) live off the herbivores. Adapting to life on the savannah has resulted in major differences between our primate cousins and us. Our stomachs are not as big as they are designed to digest smaller but more concentrated meals, rather than copious amounts of vegetation such as leaves and fruits that primates have to chomp through. We lack fur and are unique in having an effective cooling system in the form of sweat glands. Our brains, however, are larger which allowed the development of strategies for capturing prey, which may have been stronger or faster than us. It was only the consumption of animal-based fat and, in particular, a special type of fat called DHA from bone marrow and fish, which enabled the human brain to increase in size. Had we been predominantly vegetarian we might never have moved out of the trees. Bipedalism, or walking on two legs, provided a wider visual range across the savannah, leaving the hands free to use a weapon or carry food. The lack of fur, combined with the effective cooling system (sweating, as I said), enabled humans to run vast distances in hot weather. As other animals slowed down in the heat of the day, humans were able to stay alert and take advantage of those animals that had become sluggish.

Scientists have studied the comparative sizes of the brains of humans and animals. The ratio between body and brain size follows what is called 'Kleiber's Law' and enables scientists to predict brain size based on body mass.[2] However, humans were found to have brains that were massively bigger than would have been expected given the comparative smallness of their bodies. This is why our brains have such a high demand for energy – energy which is dependent upon a good intake of meat and fat, and which could not be supplied by a predominantly plant-based diet.

So successful was the hunter-gatherer way of life that we were able to migrate from the African plains and colonise most parts of the globe. This period was known as the Paleolithic Era, and later gave way to the Neolithic Era when agriculture and arable farming were introduced for the first time. That was when our problems began. Not only did we lose stature, strength and stamina, but we also became territorial and competition for resources and land ownership entered our consciousness and soon led to war. Moreover, anthropological evidence has shown that it wasn't only our skeletons that were diminishing in size. The human brain also started to shrink 10,000 years ago, making our brains 8 per cent smaller than those of our Paleo ancestors. The modern trend away from meat and fat, whilst increasing the ratio of plant-based foods in our diet, is likely to be expediting this process.

The hunter-gatherer lifestyle had much to recommend it. Hunting encouraged social interaction and a sense of community, and hunter-gatherers only worked a few hours per day, including house building, weaving and so on, leaving considerably more leisure time than we can hope for nowadays. In some ways the hunter-gatherer diet was also more diverse. Today the range of foods we select from is restricted to around 20 species of plants and animals, whilst the hunter-gatherer could choose from over 100. The diversity of available foods continues to dwindle as mass production encourages the cultivation of only a narrow range of fruits and vegetables, thus further limiting our choices, and leading to the possible extinction of some less common species. Few people realise that there exist over 100 different types of apple in the UK, but only four or five species at most can be found in the modern supermarket. Once a species has become extinct it is lost forever and it is sad that this is happening for purely commercial reasons. The spread of monoculture has implications for our countryside and heritage as well as our health, and this is discussed in chapter 10.

Even more surprising is the fact that hunter-gatherers ate a greater quantity of food than the average American – and that is no mean achievement. Nevertheless, they have been shown to have been lean and muscular, with a lower body fat ratio compared with modern man. Upon the introduction of grains into the diet, however, people became shorter, developed cavities in their teeth, died younger and started to suffer from obesity *for the first time in recorded history*. However, if a hunter-gatherer baby survived the first two years of life, his chances of surviving beyond 80 were many, many times greater than today.

Our Paleo ancestors enjoyed good health until death without the need for retirement homes. After all, a nomad had to be fit enough to keep on the move, and this included the elderly who weren't pushed around in wheelchairs or clutching on to zimmer frames. In fact, physical prowess seemed to improve with age, probably as a result of decades of exercise – not the short bursts you may engage in down at the gym, but as a way of life. Today, due to the demands of earning a living exercise tends to drop off after leaving school and physical prowess peaks in childhood – if at all.

Until recently people had eaten the food they were designed to eat for millions of years without the intervention of technology, processing or the addition of chemicals. In fact, they even managed to grow crops without pesticides – amazing. Sadly, much of what many people consume today is not food at all but consists instead of a concoction of chemicals. 'Fortified' breakfast cereals, in which synthetic vitamins and minerals in ratios that would not be found in nature, frequently provide the first carb hit of the day and set the body up for see-sawing blood sugar, cravings and fatigue. The SAD, or Standard American Diet, which consists mostly of processed, additive-laden carbs, trans-fats and factory-farmed meat, is producing a population that is both malnourished and obese. Sadly, the SAD is catching on in the UK. We may be in the 21st century when it comes to technology, but our bodies and our genes are almost the same as they were in primitive times. We really are cavemen living in an urban environment.

It is reasonable to assume that you are reading this book because you are interested in health. Hopefully, you enjoy food too. However, you may be starting to feel a little alarmed at the prospect of cutting out grains, dairy, beans and sugar as your favourite meals start to disappear off the menu. Well, that was the motivation behind my developing the Urban Caveman diet. The Urban Caveman diet differs from a strict Paleo diet as it includes foods that would not have been available in Paleo times which would look and taste familiar to us today. Much of it is cooked, and no bugs or grubs are included! Gluten is replaced by gum or seeds in bread making – although yeast is used – and breads are made in bread-making machines. Natural sweeteners that don't spike the blood sugar, low-carb breads, cakes, ice-creams and mock cheeses mean that Paleo-style eating does not have to be boring or deprive you of the tastes and textures you love.

A completely dairy-free diet can be unappealing and may not be healthy, as raw dairy is a great source of saturated fat and the vitamins A, D, K and E – vitamins that are widely deficient today partly because of the popularity of low-fat foods. Butter rarely presents a problem, even in those who are dairy intolerant, but if it does, ghee, goat or sheep butters are usually a satisfactory alternative. Egg yolks are often well tolerated too as it is often the egg whites which provoke an allergic reaction. Cheese substitutes can be made from coconut milk, and ice-cream from coconut cream. The replacement of wheat flour by coconut flour in cakes and biscuits makes them high in fibre and low in starch, and free-range eggs provide an easily digested source of nutrients, including protein, and healthy fats.

# Chapter 2

# Cereal killers

## The big breakfast

When it comes to cereals, us Brits can out-eat the Americans! Crunching our way through six kilos of breakfast cereals per person per year, which is one-and-a-half kilos more than our friends across the Pond, the British cereal market is worth a jaw-dropping £1.55 billion. Twelve million loaves of bread are eaten each day in the UK, which means that the average person gets through around 43 loaves per year. Most of us begin the day with a bowl of cereal or toast, so it is not surprising that most people assume that cereals have always been a major staple of the British diet.

However, prior to the Industrial Revolution grains were largely reserved for livestock. Bread was obviously eaten, but not in the quantities it is consumed today. It was also completely different from the modern supermarket loaf. Before the invention of the combine harvester, wheat was allowed to grow several metres tall enabling its roots to penetrate deep into the nutrient-rich soil. It would also sprout upon exposure to dew, making it more digestible and increasing its nutrient content. After having been ground into flour, it was then usually fermented into a sourdough, a process that partially digests the starches and reduces levels of the anti-nutrient called phytic acid, about which more later (see page 18). Fermentation is a process in which yeasts activate enzymes that break down the flour when added to water. Sprouting and fermentation made it possible for us to eat grass, a food for which ruminants have two stomachs. The immature, unfermented raw flour used in modern bread making has contributed to the bowel problems and gluten intolerance we see today. The genetic engineering of wheat, that final nail in the coffin of post-Paleo health, was not introduced until the middle of the 20th century, although hybridisation experiments are known to have started long before.

## It's a no-grainer

We have been led to believe that whole grains are a nutritious food and a good source of fibre, important for gut health. (Grains include wheat, rye, barley, oats, rice, millet, corn, amarynth and fibre.) However, closer examination shows that they are inferior to vegetables, seafoods, meat and fruit on both counts.[1] The devil, as they say, is in the detail. Dr Loren Cordain, the world's foremost researcher into Paleo nutrition, compared the fibre content of refined and whole grains to fruits and non-starchy vegetables.[2] He found that vegetables far outstripped grains by providing a whacking 185 grams per 1,000-calorie serving compared with refined cereals with only six grams. Fruits were the second best source of fibre, coming in at 41 grams, whilst whole grains fared only a little better than refined at 24 grams. With the exception of oats, fruits and vegetables contain more soluble fibre, which can also have a cholesterol lowering effect. And that is not all.

The average calcium content of whole grains is around 15 times lower than that of vegetables. Moreover, the calcium in vegetables is better assimilated and, since the calcium-lowering effects of grains are dose-dependent, the more grains you eat the lower your calcium status becomes. This was powerfully demonstrated by a study on infants which found that blood calcium levels took a nose-dive upon the introduction of bran.[3]

So, by replacing grains with vegetables, a grain-free diet actually increases dietary fibre and boosts mineral levels.

## The great grain robbery

The reason grains are at the bottom of the league when it comes to mineral status is due to the presence of the previously mentioned anti-nutrient called phytic acid. Since phytic acid prevents minerals from being absorbed, simply measuring the mineral content of grains would not give you the full picture. Minerals carry a positive charge and are attracted to the negatively charged gut wall where they line up awaiting transportation into the body. Unfortunately, phytic acid is a bit of a heavy weight when it comes to negative charges, and exerts a magnetic attraction so strong that it binds up the minerals before they even reach the gut wall. Like a sort of pied piper of minerals, phytic acid hoovers them up, forming compounds called phytates which then disappear out of the body in the stool.

This is the reason mineral levels decline exponentially in relation to the amount of grain eaten and why a reduction in stature of about six inches, or 15 centimetres, coincided with their introduction into the diet at the end of the Paleolithic period. Tooth decay, overcrowding of teeth, jaw problems, arthritis and degenerative diseases are almost exclusively confined to grain-eating populations. According to Dr Dietrich Kinghardt, the jaw is the first bone in the body to become demineralised,[4] and transmandibular joint (TMJ) pain, clicking and other jaw problems occur as the jaw bone runs out of minerals, predominantly zinc. Dr Nicolas Campos, an American chiropractor, claims that in the US TMJ problems affect a staggering 25 per cent of the population.

Obvious signs of low mineralisation may include brittle nails, thin hair, jaw deformities, over-crowded teeth, back and joint problems and hypermobility or double jointedness. However, mineral deficiencies have the potential to wreak havoc anywhere in the body. For example, it is known that some heart attacks are caused by cramping of the heart muscle – a problem linked to magnesium deficiency. To make matters worse, we are today exposed to environmental pollutants which exert their toxic effects by displacing minerals in enzymes, organs, bones and joints, thus further increasing our need for them. Not a great situation when you consider that white flour, rice and other grains have had an average of 80 per cent of their minerals removed by the refining process. It is now apparent to many researchers that almost everyone in the civilised world suffers from the lethal combination of nutritional deficiencies and chronic toxicity. Realisation of this could revolutionise modern medicine.

Grains have become problematic over the last few decades because of changes in the way they are grown and prepared. Coeliac disease, in which bowel symptoms arise after ingestion of gluten, is thought to affect one in 100 people in the UK. Young people today are five times more likely to have the disease compared with young people in the 1950s. According to Coeliac UK, only 10 to 15 per cent of sufferers are actually diagnosed, so sensitivity to gluten is likely to be a far greater problem than is realised. Whilst doctors still rely upon biopsy to make a diagnosis of coeliac, it is now recognised that antibodies to gluten (transglutaminase and anti-gliadin) may be present in the blood even in the absence of bowel symptoms.[5] Coeliac disease is rapidly being recognised as the tip of the gluten iceberg, with problems ranging from cross-reactivity, in which gluten stimulates intolerances to other foods, to autoimmune diseases. Modern gluten, bred to be more, well, glutenous, is difficult to digest and levels have increased by 50 per cent in the modern loaf over the past 50 years. This is compounded by a lack of dietary cholesterol and fat soluble vitamins in infancy, resulting in inadequate development of our digestive systems.[6]

However, not all hunter-gatherer diets were grain-free.

Californian Indians, considered the most 'primitive' of Native Americans, have been consuming wild grains and high starch root vegetables for more than 100,000 years.[7] Arabic nations, where gluten sensitivity is rare, have a long tradition of eating wheat. Grains were traditionally soaked, sprouted or fermented into sourdoughs which not only partially digests the starches but which also significantly reduces phytic acid levels. Wild grains prepared in this way are often better tolerated, although a period of abstinence of around 18 months to two years may be necessary if you have already become sensitised. After this time you may be able to reintroduce grains on a rotational basis, starting with properly prepared wild grains. Treatments to colonise the gut with healthy bacteria, to boost secretory IgA levels and to strengthen gut wall integrity help reduce sensitivity and improve immunity. All grains contain gluten, but it is the type of gluten found in wheat, rye, barley and some oats that presents the greatest problem.

### The corn maze

Many turn to corn as a replacement for wheat but corn, in common with all grains, contains gluten. Although different from that found in wheat, rye, some oats and barley, there is very little known about corn gluten. Corn is generally poorly tolerated by those sensitive to wheat as it too is high in indigestible starches. Unfortunately, removing only wheat or gluten is rarely the answer. Damage to the gut from any grain will make it nigh on impossible to digest any complex carbohydrate and the diet may need to be limited to simple sugars such as those found in non-starchy vegetables until the gut is healed.

The problem with corn is not limited to its gluten or starch content. Second to soy, it is the most genetically modified food on the planet. High in calories and low in nutrients, corn is a comparatively new food and is routinely being fed to animals, including cows and fish, and is then indirectly ingested by humans. You may be surprised to learn that cows and fish are not natural corn eaters, and this is why farm animals fed corn have a shorter lifespan. Unlike grass-fed beef, corn-fed beef is linked to heart disease, diabetes, cancer and obesity. Corn also contains a type of sugar called fructose which is toxic to the liver. Both fructose and alcohol look the same to the liver, being metabolised in the same way and producing the same metabolites. Furthermore, corn syrup, which is often added to processed foods, is contaminated with mercury. Corn has been shown to stimulate inflammation in coeliacs who fail to realise that gluten is just the most obvious part of a wider problem.

Since the introduction of GM corn, evidence of toxicity has emerged linking it to gluten sensitivity. Eighty-eight per cent of the world's corn is now genetically modified. A study in the *Journal of Applied Toxicology* found that Bt toxin which is added to GM corn is not only resistant to digestion but actually damages gut cells, provoking gluten intolerance and autoimmune diseases. Gluten sensitivity is escalating in the US with a third of the population now having been diagnosed whilst many others struggle with irritable bowel, migraines, mood disorders and other unpleasant symptoms. Intolerance to gluten is commonly found in autism and the rise of autism by 250 per cent in the GM-sodden US directly parallels the rise of GM foods like corn in the food chain.

### Rice takes

Rice is assumed to be a benign grain. However, its high starch content of 80 per cent in brown, rising to 85.8 per cent in white, combined with its sticky, glutinous consistency after cooking, make it very difficult to digest. Stimulating an excessive output of pancreatic enzymes to break down the sugars whilst providing as little as 5 per cent protein, brown rice is not quite the health food it has been cracked up to be. Furthermore, its glue-like consistency and high sugar content could result in fermentation in a gut struggling to process it. This is why gas, bloating and sleepiness often follow its consumption. Sharing top billing with grains like wheat in the phytic acid stakes, and with its low mineral status (1 per cent calcium, 2 per cent iron and 10 per cent magnesium), rice is nutritionally inferior to vegetables and could even cause loss of more nutrients than it provides. Containing only 5 per cent protein and upwards of 80 per cent starch, rice would not be a wise choice if blood sugar or weight were an issue. Often assumed to be high in fibre, one cup of brown rice contains 3.5 grams of fibre compared with 5 grams in an unpeeled apple and 8.36 grams in a cup of raspberries.

## Other grain issues

Unlike meat and fish, no grain contains the full complement of amino acids (proteins) and they are also low in fat. Those fats they do contain come with an unhealthy ratio of omega-6 to omega-3. Furthermore, since grains contain no vitamin A (or D), night blindness, infection and stunted growth are more prevalent amongst grain-eating populations. Also reported are deficiencies in vitamin B1 (thiamine) and B3 (niacin), both of which are damaged by the milling process, whilst the B vitamin biotin is almost non-existent in grains. This is unfortunate since biotin is needed to metabolise carbohydrates but is often found to be deficient in grain eaters. Nor do grains contain vitamin C, but because both biotin and vitamin C are used up when digesting them, they can cause what is known in the nutrition trade as 'negative nutrition'. In other words, nutrients are needed from other sources in order to metabolise grains.

Grains, in common with fizzy drinks, contain excessive levels of the mineral phosphorus. Whilst phosphorus is needed for calcium metabolism, both phosphorus and calcium have to be kept within a narrow ratio. If the phosphorus to calcium ratio becomes too high, it will interfere with protein metabolism, and this can result in the breakdown of muscle to provide energy. Converting protein released from muscles into glucose is an inefficient way of producing energy, and this is one of the reasons why energy improves when you give up grains. Grain-eating can reverse the calcium/phosphorus ratio by pushing up phosphorus levels whilst calcium is lost in the stool in the form of a phytate. Everyone knows that calcium is important for bones and teeth, but less well known is its role in nervous system function, where lack of calcium can contribute to anxiety and insomnia.

Grain (and dairy) consumption can plunge the body into calcium imbalance in which calcium becomes *bio-unavailable* due to lack of co-factors, such as the other minerals and vitamins needed for its uptake. When this happens the thyroid gland can become imbalanced as calcium and potassium respectively slow and stimulate the gland. Unused calcium can become a menace, ending up being deposited along artery walls or formed into stones in the gall bladder or kidneys. Calcium balance in grain eaters will be further compromised if magnesium is low, which it invariably is, because without magnesium, calcium becomes useless.

## Grains and hormones

Vitamin D behaves more like a hormone than a vitamin because it affects cells and organs throughout the body. Essential for calcium metabolism and immune function, vitamin D has been the subject of a great deal of research over the last decade which continues to reveal how crucial it is for health. However, it has been estimated that 95 per cent of us in northern latitudes could be deficient in it. This is partly due to lack of sunlight, but our old friend wheat has to bear some of the responsibility as well.

Wheat contains a **lectin**[8] (a special type of protein) called

WGA or 'wheat germ agglutinin'. Lectins can create all sorts of problems as they bind up sugars and block the carbohydrate receptors on red blood cells. They are found in all foods and are usually harmless because they are unable to cross the intestinal barrier and gain entry into the body. However, WGA has no trouble crossing the gut wall. Once in the bloodstream it does what its name implies and causes 'agglutination', or clumping, of red blood cells, thus increasing the risk of clots. By docking on to their carbohydrate receptors – in which red blood cells are abundant – WGA can then hitch-hike around the body and this is where the fun starts.

Lectins are nothing if not opportunistic, and like the Del-boy of foreign proteins, they never miss a chance. They also attach themselves to receptors for the blood sugar hormone, insulin. Hormones are a bit like a key that fits into the cell lock but if lectins have got there first hormones like insulin won't get a look in. Instead of carrying glucose into cells insulin then remains locked in the blood stream causing what is known as hyperinsulinaemia. They say the devil makes work for idle hands, and redundant insulin will always find something else to do. In women this usually means stimulating the ovaries leading to polycystic ovarian syndrome, whilst in men it may lower testosterone, causing impotence, and in both sexes it can cause inflammation, poor blood sugar regulation and disease.

Once joy-riding around the body, WGA can hop off at any point and penetrate any cell it chooses. It is the bully-boy of lectins, bypassing the gut wall, elbowing sugars and hormones out of red blood cells before muscling-in to what is called the 'nuclear pore', which is where the action is, hormonally speaking. (The nuclear pore is a bit like a nuclear bouncer deciding what goes in and what comes out of the nucleus.) Hormones work by attaching to the nuclear pore in order to stimulate cellular activity. Different cells have different jobs to do but they await directions from hormones so that their activity can be modified according to need. However, if WGA has gate-crashed the hormonal party and assumed squatters' rights, real hormones are prevented from working, and we can only guess at the confused instructions WGA may be imparting.

Since vitamin D acts more like a hormone in the body, it too can come under the spell of WGA, and this is why chronic vitamin D deficiency is often found in wheat-eaters. WGA can incapacitate vitamin D in the same way it incapacitates other hormones. Vitamin D is needed for immunity, but since lectins also disrupt immune function and shrink the thymus, the gland that conducts the immune system orchestra, eating wheat regularly may increase the risk of infections and allergies.

## Coeliac disease – the tip of the gluten iceberg

Despite modern research implicating gluten in hundreds of health problems, including autism, dementia, Addison's disease, schizophrenia, eating disorders, migraines, bipolar disorder, mental health disorders, irritable bowel syndrome, thyroid diseases, and infertility,[9] current medical dogma recognises only coeliac disease and, at a pinch, dermatitis herpetiformis as being caused by gluten intolerance. Even so, it was a decades-long struggle to get gluten's role in coeliac disease recognised at all. Previously attributed to malabsorption and problems digesting fat, it wasn't until the 1930s when Dr Dicke discovered that a wheat-free diet resulted in remission of symptoms, that the role of diet was even considered. Unfortunately, the link between diet and digestive problems still eludes many gastroenterologists today. Nevertheless, it took a further 20 years for this heretical concept to take hold as grains were considered a healthy food, so it was not until the 1960s, when tissue biopsies were developed, that coeliac disease was finally conceded as being caused by gluten sensitivity. They got there in the end! Or did they?

New research has shown that nowadays the majority of

patients with gluten intolerance suffer no digestive symptoms at all, but are more likely to present with mental health problems or autoimmune diseases. Recently, a new clinical entity has emerged known as 'non-coeliac gluten sensitivity'; although other factors in wheat have also been found to be problematic, so this too may be a misnomer. It is as if with each subsequent generation the problems caused by gluten are penetrating more deeply into the body. Dr Thomas O'Bryan, an authority on gluten sensitivity, estimates that for every person diagnosed with coeliac disease, there are at least another eight suffering from gluten-induced conditions that go unrecognised. The families of diagnosed coeliacs have been shown to produce antibodies in response to eating gluten *even though they do not suffer from the disease itself*, but often have related problems currently dipping below the gluten radar.

Conservative estimates state that over 2 million Americans suffer from coeliac disease,[10] but since 80 per cent remain undiagnosed the actual figure could be truly staggering. This may be partly due to ignorance, but also because gut biopsy is not the most reliable method of obtaining a diagnosis. In order for a positive diagnosis to be obtained, gluten has to have been eaten over a two-week period prior to biopsy and if the tissue sample is taken from a part of the gut that is not affected, a false negative will be obtained. Understandably, many people, reluctant to go back to the gluten-induced misery of coeliac, choose to forgo the test.

Meanwhile, some independent laboratories are developing more sophisticated antibody assays to help identify gluten sensitivities unrelated to coeliac disease. It takes dogged persistence to obtain a diagnosis of the condition, necessitating an average of six visits to different doctors over nearly a decade, so it is not surprising that under 20 per cent ever get picked up. Dr Fasano, who directs the Center for Celiac Research at the University of Maryland School of Medicine, believes that gluten sensitivity has now reached epidemic proportions, affecting more than 20 million Americans – which is bad news for a nation fed from the prairies.

## Mi-grain and other diseases linked to gluten

Beloved of bakers, gluten is the protein that gives bread its elasticity. Difficult to replicate, its absence in gluten-free baking is responsible for the cement-like consistency of many alternative breads on the market today. Similar in structure to the milk protein casein that gives cheese its stretchy texture, gluten (and casein) can behave rather like chewing gum in the gut, stimulating the production of mucous and generally bunging up the works and preventing nutrient absorption. Like WGA, gluten (and casein) can permeate the intestinal barrier, running rings round the immune system and causing trouble throughout the body. Since cross reactivity between similar foods has now been recognised, and gluten and casein are broken down by the same enzyme, DPP-1V or 'dipeptidyl-peptidase', it seems obvious that coeliacs almost certainly need to eliminate dairy produce as well.

## The grain brain drain

The effects of gluten on the brain have been highlighted by a number of studies around the world. Dr Thomas O'Bryan quotes research in which lesions detected by MRI scans in patients with migraine or dementia lessened or disappeared within a year after switching to a gluten-free diet. In the book *Human Brain and Health and Disease*, Dr Stephen Gislason writes of the link between the opioid effects on the brain of gluten and casein in autism and allied diseases. He also found an increased incidence of depression amongst adolescents with wheat sensitivity. Other symptoms often linked to gluten intolerance include sleep disturbances, mood instability, memory loss, irritability and impaired cognition.

A trial carried out as part of the Stanley Research Programme at Sheppard Pratt, Baltimore, in February 2011 revealed an increased prevalence of antibodies to **gliadin** (a protein in wheat) in patients with bipolar disorder. There are studies going back decades confirming the link between schizophrenia and gluten sensitivity including one at the Johns Hopkins School of Medicine, also part of the Stanley Research Programme, which identified antibodies to gliadin in schizophrenics that were only slightly different from the antibodies to gliadin found in coeliacs.

ADHD has long been associated with diet, and a 12-month Italian study of 132 coeliacs aged between three and 57 years at the Regional Hospital in Bolzana discovered that the adoption of a gluten-free diet resulted in a substantial improvement in ADHD scores. A paper published in the *Journal of Attention Disorders* in November 2006 stated: '…a large number with untreated coeliac may show signs of ADHD…' In a country that gave the world pizza and pasta, that must have come as a blow to many Italians.

Even in the absence of antibodies to gluten, there is no doubt that most people experience improved memory and better concentration, and feel more alert, when following a wheat-free diet. Leaving aside the possible immunological and opioid reactions to wheat which can impair mood and cognition, the reduction in available nutrients that result from eating grains is bound to have a negative effect on brain function. In the book *Nutritional Balancing* by Dr Lawrence Wilson,[11] specific mineral imbalances are shown to be predictive of mood and behaviour, with a correlation between the presence of toxic metals and criminality.

Unless engaged in exercise, the brain has a greater demand for glucose and other nutrients than the rest of the body put together. This is why zinc deficiency and poor blood sugar regulation have a direct impact on sleep, mood, behaviour and cognition. We have already seen that WGA, the lectin found in wheat, can inhibit glucose transportation, and we know that when glucose levels drop, with the exception of the cortex, the brain starts to shut down. The signs that this is happening can include poor concentration, anxiety and irritability – a normal state for some people today.

A dip in blood sugar also accounts for the drowsiness that can overwhelm us after a lunch of sandwiches or pasta – a phenomenon reported by teachers attempting to teach their semi-comatose charges in the afternoon. Incidentally, the only part of the brain to remain functional when there is a shortage of nutrients is the pre-frontal cortex, the part associated with aggression. An ancient survival mechanism that enabled us to defend ourselves if starving, its modern counterpart is more likely to manifest as road rage or violence. In Yorkshire, England, adolescent males were spared custodial sentences when it was demonstrated that their crimes had been committed at a time when they had been hypoglycaemic – that is, low in blood sugar.

## Wheats of engineering

The genetic engineering of wheat has almost certainly driven the increase in mental and emotional problems seen today. Proteins altered by selective breeding are frequently not recognised as a food by our immune systems. Genetically weakened by agricultural breeding practices, modern grains bear no resemblance to those found in the wild.[12] Spelt and kamut, ancient forms of wheat which are sometimes better tolerated, still come with all the disadvantages associated with grains, and an immune system primed to react to wheat will react to unadulterated grains as well. Symptoms associated with the new high-gluten wheats include bloating, fluid-retention, joint stiffness, headaches, migraines, asthma, indigestion, constipation, sweet cravings, poor cognition and sluggishness, and are often alleviated upon adopting a gluten-free/dairy-free diet.

Modern wheat contains roughly 50 per cent more gluten than it did only five decades ago. To add insult to injury, genetic engineering has made modern gluten even more indigestible. As I have mentioned, gluten gives dough its stretchy consistency, and genetically modified gluten makes it possible to bake bigger loaves from less wheat by filling them with air, but this is not something you would want to fill your gut with. When gluten hits the intestine it can be extremely tenacious, adhering to the intestinal wall like, as I have said before, bubble gum. Eating whole wheat has been likened to eating razor blades because it is also abrasive and can cause the gut to bleed. In order to protect itself, the gut may produce extra mucous which can, over time, harden into what is called 'mucoid plaque', and this can solidify along the gut wall, interfering with digestion and nutrient uptake. Lining the gut wall like an oil slick, it also makes it practically impossible for beneficial bacteria to gain a foothold. It is estimated that many of us are carrying several pounds of solidified mucous and trapped faecal matter around with us.

Nonetheless, over the last 200 years, grains have risen to supremacy and have now become the staple food of the Western world. Only 50 years ago evils like mass-produced breakfast cereals had yet to be unleashed on a population that had been accustomed to starting the day with bacon and eggs, and pasta had hardly found its way out of Italy. Nowadays, grains are invariably eaten at almost every meal, with cereal and toast for breakfast, sandwiches for lunch, and pasta, rice or pastry for dinner.

## Gut out grains

Grains are not a very efficient food to produce, requiring technological intervention, such as milling, fermenting, sprouting, soaking or cooking to make them edible. To overcome the problems of digesting them, our predecessors used first to soak or ferment them over several days, and even then they were only eaten in moderation and never raw as they are today.

Grain consumption is a major contributory factor in the

development of **leaky gut syndrome**, which sets the stage for autoimmune diseases. This is a condition in which the gut wall becomes too porous, allowing leakage of incompletely digested foods into the body. You may think this might improve nutrient absorption, but sadly the opposite is true, as a damaged gut wall cannot effectively transport nutrients into the body. The risk of allergies is also increased with leaky gut syndrome, as, unable to recognise an incompletely digested food, the immune system will often mount an antibody attack instead. Thump first and ask questions later.

The reason autoimmune diseases such as rheumatoid arthritis and type 2 diabetes are linked with non-Paleo foods is that they contain proteins that are almost identical to those of our own body tissues. If the immune system fails to differentiate between a food protein and a body protein, its own tissues will also come under fire, which is likely to be why autoimmune diseases first started to appear after the Industrial Revolution.

## Grains – high maintenance and low return

Despite the claims of vegetarians, only about 11 per cent of the earth's surface is suitable for grain production, whereas animals can graze on sparse, inhospitable land. Grains are also quite energy expensive to produce as they are small and difficult to harvest. The seeds need to be separated from the plant, which is time-consuming and requires more energy than the grain itself can provide, and this would certainly not have appealed to our Stone Age ancestors who downed tools after only three-hours![12]

## Pesticides and grains

Grains are also a dirty food.[13] There is a deep groove in wheat that cannot be cleaned and this often gets infested with insect droppings, and urine and hair from rats and mice, necessitating the use of insecticides and fungicides. There is a high-microbe content in grains, so protectants (such as chlorpyrifos-methyl and pyrethrins) are used to kill them off. Therefore all non-organic grains are contaminated with pesticides which can damage the liver and brain. They are also fumigated with methyl-bromide (which blocks iodine uptake needed to make thyroid hormone), aluminium phosphide and magnesium phosphide. Part of the fumigation process involves exposing the grain to high temperatures which also damage the protein content, especially the gluten, which is another reason why modern gluten is particularly difficult to digest.

## Whole grains for *hell*th?

As Dr Cordain states in *The Paleo Answer*,[14] government recommendations to eat a diet predominantly based on whole grains whilst minimising meat and fat consumption fly in the face of all the evidence. If modern wheat is toxic for a significant percentage of the population, it cannot possibly be promoted as the cornerstone of a healthy diet. In view of the irrefutable case the prosecution is mounting against wheat, this advice is unhelpful if not downright dangerous for the majority of people. It is to be hoped that the whole grain dogma that has influenced modern health policies may soon be revoked, but I am not optimistic. Although elimination of gluten and grains is becoming more commonplace amongst the health conscious, there is still a long way to go before there is official condemnation of current health guidelines. Rather than waiting for an expert to tell them what their bodies already know, for increasing numbers the verdict on gluten has already been passed. Grains are inexpensive and convenient to mass produce and transport. Removing them from their primary position in the modern diet would have serious and far-reaching economic ramifications. Bear this in mind next time you see the main-stream media, or a medic, pushing the whole-grain, low-fat diet and telling you to cut down on red meat.

## Quick recap

- Vegetables contain more fibre than wheat.
- Vegetables provide more calcium than wheat.
- Grains contain phytic acid which can cause minerals to be lost from the body.
- Grains don't contain the full complement of amino acids.

## Personal health check

### *Could you be low in minerals?*

Tick any of the following that apply to you:

| | | | |
|---|---|---|---|
| | Brittle hair or nails | | Jaw problems |
| | Overcrowded teeth | | Muscle cramps or stiffness |
| | Clench jaw when asleep | | Back problems |
| | Tinnitus (ringing in ears) | | Fillings in teeth |
| | Double-jointed | | Women only: sweet craving before periods (sign of low magnesium) |
| | Sweet cravings | | History of gall or kidney stones |
| | White marks on 3 or more nails | | Stretch marks (sign of low zinc) |

## *Could you be sensitive to gluten?*

Tick any of the following that apply to you or members of your family. These symptoms could also be due to other causes, but if you tick several boxes it might be worth trying a gluten-free diet.

| | | | |
|---|---|---|---|
| | Addictions (food, drugs, alcohol) | | Autism, chronic fatigue, eating disorders, behavioural problems or learning difficulties |
| | Migraine | | Mental health problems |
| | Bloating, wind or irritable bowel | | Autoimmune disease |
| | Depression or bipolar disorder | | Food cravings |
| | Would find it hard to give up bread | | Sleepy after meals containing wheat |
| | Fluid retention | | Sluggishness and low energy |
| | Constipation or constipation alternating with loose stools | | Hormonal problems |
| | Stiffness/muscle aches | | Brain fog |

# Chapter 3

# Milking the facts about dairy

When asked the question, 'How do you know our hunter-gatherer ancestors didn't drink milk?',[1] Dr Loren Cordain, researcher into Paleo nutrition, asks his audience whether anyone has ever tried to approach a wild animal, let alone attempted to milk it. Nevertheless, drinking milk is perceived as healthy and natural, although humans are the only species who consume milk beyond infancy. After the age of about three, around 70 per cent of us lack the enzymes to digest it.

Cow's milk is ideal for calves, who require a nutritionally dense food high in hormones to promote fast growth. Humans, on the other hand, are often completely helpless until their 20s. Calves reach adulthood in only 18 months so high levels of calcium are required to meet this demand. Cow's milk is therefore significantly higher in calcium providing 120 milligrams per 100 millilitres (mg/ml) compared with breast milk which has only 34 mg/100 ml. The hypercalcaemia (high calcium in the blood) that can result from drinking cow's milk is one of the reasons that feeding it to humans – who require 21 years (and longer in some cases!) to reach maturity – can have serious consequences for health.

There has long been an association between milk consumption and cardio-vascular disease,[2] and this is partly due to its lactose (sugar) content. Lactose is made of two sugars, glucose and galactose, which need to be separated by an enzyme called 'lactase', but this is the enzyme that most of us lose around the age of three. Yoghurt, however, is low in lactose as it is broken down by lactose-fermenting bacteria, giving it its sour taste.

How do we know that milk-drinking is detrimental to health? Well, until about 25 years ago the standard treatment for stomach ulcers was to drink lots of milk. Based on the belief that ulcers were caused by an over-abundance of acid, the sufferer was drinking more milk than a newborn baby. Known as the 'Sippy Diet', milk was promoted for its neutralising effect on stomach acid until two Australian researchers identified bacterial infection with *Helicobacter pylori* as being the cause of ulcers. What is of interest to us is that of those who adhered to the milk-drinking protocol, 42 per cent died of fatal heart attacks.[3] Since 1989, several papers have reported a direct link between milk consumption and cardiovascular disease *which has been found to be greater than that of any other food.*[4]

## Milk marketing fraud

The RDA, or 'Recommended Daily Allowance' for nutrients, is set at levels regarded by nutritionists as woefully inadequate. Commonly referred to as 'Ridiculous Daily Arbitraries', RDAs are just high enough to prevent overt deficiency diseases, but nowhere near sufficient to optimise health and function. Consider, then, that the calcium intake of the hunter-gatherer diet falls short of the modern RDA by 30 per cent. The successful marketing of milk as a source of calcium has firmly established dairy produce in the minds of many as necessary for the prevention of diseases like rickets and osteoporosis. It may therefore come as a surprise to learn that osteoporosis is almost exclusively confined to populations who consume milk.

Whilst it is true that milk is high in calcium, it is low in the nutrients needed to make it available to the body. Without vitamins D and K, and the minerals magnesium and boron, calcium is largely unusable. This may explain why stone formation, artherosclerosis, arthritis and cardiovascular disease have a proven association with high calcium levels as the body has to dump it somewhere. An inability to utilise calcium, which tends to affect populations consuming dairy, causes symptoms of both excess and deficiency. This is why calcium supplementation is rarely necessary. In fact, calcium supplementation can actually make things worse.

Magnesium, a mineral protective against heart disease, needs to be kept in balance with calcium. Since calcium raises insulin levels whilst magnesium lowers them, a high ratio of calcium to magnesium can upset blood sugar regulation and contribute to high blood insulin and the development of type 2 diabetes. Levels of magnesium in milk are comparatively low at 11 milligrams per 100 millilitres, with calcium being around 121 milligrams per 100 millilitres, giving milk an unhealthy ratio of 12:1 calcium to magnesium. This is why milk-drinkers almost invariably suffer from magnesium deficiency. This ratio is almost double what it should be and way off that of the hunter-gatherer, which was around 2:1 or 1:1.

Leafy green vegetables are a good source of magnesium. Strawberries are high in boron. Both these minerals are essential for calcium uptake. Unfortunately, almost everyone on the standard Western diet is deficient in magnesium due to the combined effects of phytic acid (see chapter 2, page 18) and the low magnesium to calcium ratio found in cow's milk. Sheep and goats milks have slightly better ratios, but are still not ideal.

In fact, all the mineral ratios in cow's milk scream its unsuitability for humans. Minerals tend to work in pairs alternately stimulating and inhibiting function in different parts of the body, enabling it to adapt to changing demands for energy and rest. For example, magnesium slows the adrenals down whilst sodium stimulates them, so the modern diet, with its high intake of sodium and lack of magnesium, could contribute to increased anxiety and a trigger-happy stress response. Unsurprisingly, with 100 millilitres of milk providing 43 millgrams of sodium and only 11 milligrams of magnesium, the sodium to magnesium ratio of cow's milk also falls wide of the mark.

This pattern is repeated with regard to the thyroid gland since calcium puts the brakes on and potassium accelerates it. When these two minerals go out of balance, as they are likely to when consuming cow's milk, thyroid output could become unbalanced too. The ratio of calcium to potassium in whole milk is 1 to 1.38 respectively, which is far from the optimal ratio of 4 to 1 calcium to potassium.

Many countries, including Canada and Denmark, are now recommending that cow's milk should not be given to infants below the age of at least nine months because of its low iron content and tendency to cause rectal bleeding in babies: this latter would obviously worsen an existing iron deficiency.

## Reduce inflammation by avoiding milk

Almost every disease involves inflammation. Until the 1990s everyone *knew* that atherosclerosis was simply the result of fat and calcium clogging up the arteries and thus the customary advice was to reduce dietary fat. It is now known that atherosclerosis is initiated by inflammation causing injury to the blood vessels, to which the body then responds by plugging the wounds with cholesterol and calcium – a sort of natural Band-Aid.

Those foods implicated in inflammation include the usual suspects of grains, dairy and legumes. Dr Cordain states that milk is essentially filtered blood,[5] containing hormones, immune factors and proteins pertinent to cow physiology. Bovine insulin is different from human insulin by three proteins, whilst porcine insulin differs by only one. Antibodies to bovine insulin have been found in insulin-dependent diabetics, and although the process is incompletely understood it is thought that this may effectively immunise genetically susceptible individuals against their own insulin by a process known as **molecular mimicry**.

Another milk protein, bovine serum albumin (BSA), is almost identical to the collagen in our joints and to the pancreatic cells that produce insulin. In some, antibodies produced in response to BSA may attack the joints, causing rheumatoid arthritis, whilst in others they may attack the pancreas, resulting in insulin-dependent diabetes.

Molecular mimicry underlies all autoimmune diseases. The immune system doesn't simply 'go mad' as has long been assumed, but is actually fire-fighting in response to the continuous onslaught of foreign proteins from foods that we are not genetically equipped to eat. The immune system is primed to produce antibodies to alien invaders, and proteins from dairy, grains and legumes are definitely not part of the in-crowd. Whether proteins from ancient grains and raw dairy would have the same effect probably varies from individual to individual. In the case of atherosclerosis, the culprit is thought to be another milk protein called 'xanthine oxidase' (XO), which just happens to be found in the epithelial cells that line our arteries. It is believed that antibodies to XO may be attacking the artery walls and provoking the cascade that results in inflammation, damage and congestion known as atherosclerosis.

## Spot the white lie

Until 2002,[6] the dermatological party line was that acne was caused by hormonal fluctuations and had nothing to do with diet. Teenage girls were therefore put on the pill and both sexes were prescribed antibiotics in an attempt to suppress their acne. However, were acne to be a symptom of adolescent hormonal fluctuations then all pubescent hunter-gatherers would have been sprouting spots like their Western counterparts, but this was not the case.

Whilst it is obviously impossible to tell whether our Paleo ancestors suffered from pimples since they didn't leave any photographs behind, Dr Cordain studied two modern hunter-gatherer communities who consumed neither milk nor processed foods and, to his surprise, discovered acne to be entirely absent. His research prompted other studies, one at Harvard University and another in Australia, both of which confirmed his findings. In his book *The Paleo Answer*, Dr Cordain quotes many anecdotal examples of acne remission upon adopting the Paleo diet.

## Milk, hormones and blood sugar

A study in 2005[7] showed milk reduces our sensitivity to insulin. Twenty-four eight-year-old boys were placed on either a high-milk or high-meat diet for a week. The high-milk group demonstrated a worsening of insulin responsiveness of 100 per cent, with the entire group becoming insulin resistant within only seven days. In the meat-eating group, however, insulin sensitivity remained constant.

I have already discussed the role of hormones as growth promoters in calves (see page 35). Cow's milk naturally contains a multitude of growth hormones, such as insulin-like growth factors (IGFs), insulin-like growth factor binding proteins, growth hormone and growth hormone releasing factors, making milk the ideal food for a rapidly growing calf. However, high-production, intensively reared herds are routinely given additional growth promoters, hormones and antibiotics to increase yields, and these are then passed on to the consumer.

A number of steroidal hormones naturally occur in milk, including oestrogens, progesterone, pregnenolones, DHEA (dehydroepiandrosterone, or 'androstenolone') and testosterone, and many others produced by the pituitary gland to stimulate hormonal responses in the calf, some of which also affect blood sugar regulation. Thyroid stimulating hormones, hormones to improve calcium uptake, hormones to boost appetite and hormones to activate the immune system make milk a sort of bovine pharmacopeia – great, in moderation, for the baby calf who needs to put a growth spurt on, but possibly not so great for us. The high levels of female hormones in commercially produced milk could make it the food-equivalent of the contraceptive pill! It is likely that the recent proliferation of hormonal disorders, declining sperm counts, infertility, hormonal cancers, obesity and precocious puberty may be partly associated with excessive hormonal stimulation from drinking the milk of intensively reared cows.

A study carried out on behalf of UK clothing retailers published in 2013 has found that children aged between four and 16 years have been progressively getting bigger since measurements were last taken in 1978. Girls have grown taller by an average 3 centimetres (1 ³⁄₁₆ inches), their chest measurements have increased by 7 centimetres (2¾ inches) and their waist and hip measurements have gone up by 10 centimetres (4 inches) and 4 centimetres (1½ inches) respectively. Boys were found to be 3 centimetres (1 ³⁄₁₆ inches) taller, with chests and waists that had expanded by 9 centimetres (3 ⅝ inches) and hips that were 7 centimetres (2¾ inches) wider. So great is this problem that clothing manufacturers have had to resize their clothes to reduce the cost of processing the high percentage of returns. The report blames lack of exercise in combination with an increase in sugar intake and, whilst both these undoubtedly play a part, they cannot be held responsible for increases in height, as height is determined by hormonal stimulation. If we grew taller simply from eating sugar and lounging in front of the TV we'd all be giants!

The bigger chest size in girls was attributed to the earlier onset of puberty but this does not explain why boys' chests should also be getting bigger. What is disturbing is that whilst girls are tending to experience puberty earlier, it is becoming later in boys. It is also worrying that the boys' chest and hip sizes have increased even more than the girls', suggesting they too have undergone changes stimulated by oestrogens. Xenoestrogens (environmental oestrogens or oestrogens that are not your own) have a known feminising effect on other creatures, such as fish. If boys are developing 'man boobs' and curvy hips at adolescence, this could have serious implications for their future sexual health. Elevated oestrogen is associated with a reduced sperm count and an increased risk of prostate cancer, both of which are becoming more prevalent amongst males in the developed world.

It is known that all cancers share some degree of insulin resistance and oestrogenic stimulation. That is not to suggest that drinking cow's milk causes cancer, but its challenge to the immune system in combination with its disruption of hormonal function may tip the balance, especially when processed foods, prescription drugs and pollution are factored into the equation.

One of the proteins in milk, insulin-like growth factor (IGF), promotes growth in both healthy and cancerous tissues. Dr Cordain cites a study which found that milk raises IGF-1 in the blood, also causing insulin levels to rise.[8] This flooding of the bloodstream with insulin not only disrupts blood sugar regulation but leads to an insensitivity to insulin (**insulin resistance**, as already mentioned), which can eventually result in type 2 diabetes. Since cow's milk has been shown to raise insulin levels and given that it also contains bovine insulin, its association with blood sugar disruption is irrefutable. Over the last 40 years numerous studies have demonstrated a correlation between elevated IGF-1 and breast and prostate cancer, and a causal link between milk drinking and ovarian cancer.[9] This is not surprising since both breast and prostate cancer are often driven by high levels of oestrogen, a hormone obviously high in the milk produced by lactating cows (see below, Modern milk, page 82). The evidence suggests that we are being regularly and indirectly dosed with hormones from factory-farmed foods. Children are particularly vulnerable to the effects of hormones due to their smaller body size and reduced ability to break them down.

In order for baby calves to derive the maximum benefit from their mothers' hormones and immunological proteins, these have to survive digestion and gain access into their blood stream. Milk, in common with grains and legumes, also comes loaded with protease inhibitors which switch off protein digestion to ensure the hormones enter the body intact.[10] However, they are damaged by the high temperatures to which milk is exposed during pasteurisation, triggering an immune response in some people which can lead to the production of autoantibodies to their own natural hormones. This is what happens in lupus, for example – an autoimmune disease in which antibodies to thyroid hormones are produced that prevent it from docking onto cells.

## Milk as HRT

Several forms of oestrogen are found in milk from intensively farmed cows. To increase milk production, which begins in the latter part of pregnancy, dairy cows are artificially inseminated three months after having given birth,[11] ensuring that milk production is maintained for 305 days a year. Unfortunately, this practice dramatically increases the levels of oestrogen in the milk. Oestrogen sulphate is the preferred form, but is the same as that used to make HRT. Oestrogen sulphate has what is referred to as 'high biological activity', which means it gains easy access into the blood stream. Since oestrogens given in the birth control pill work by fooling the body into thinking it is pregnant, could excessive oestrogenic exposure from modern milk be contributing to declining sperm counts in males and infertility in women?

## Cow's milk and human digestion

The digestive system of a human is quite different from that of a cow who has extra stomachs to help process the herbivorous diet.[12] Just what happens when humans ingest milk can be demonstrated by comparison with the manufacture of white glue. Glue is made by exposing milk to acid and then removing the excess fluid. This is exactly what happens in the human stomach when drinking milk, and it can cause bloating and flatulence in some individuals, and give the stool a sticky consistency.[13] This is why milk is often linked to infantile colic. Whether ingested directly from formula or indirectly from the maternal diet via the breast, colicky babies are often reacting to proteins like gluten and casein that have resisted digestion, resulting in pain and cramping in the baby.

In the US it is now impossible to buy formula made from cow's milk as paediatricians have realised that cow's milk should not be consumed under the age of one year.[14] In the UK, however, most infant formulas are made from cow's milk that has been processed to make it 'suitable' for babies. They may also contain, among other things, soya protein, structured vegetable oils, nucleotides and fish oils, and will have undergone damaging processes like homogenisation, about which more very shortly.

Like wheat, cow's milk is also associated with **leaky gut syndrome**, which is present in nearly everyone today and underlies allergies and autoimmune diseases. The reason grains and milk are linked to seasonal allergies like hay fever is because of a process called **cross reactivity**. Cow's milk has long been implicated in hay fever and asthma and this is in part due to the fact that cows are grass eaters. Therefore, antibodies originally produced in response to milk proteins could also be triggered upon the inhalation of grasses. One study reported an improvement in asthmatic symptoms upon eliminating dairy in 82 per cent of sufferers.

One of the milk proteins, beta-casomorphin-7, which is of particular relevance in autism and allied disorders, stimulates mucous production. However, if it leaches out of the gut it can stimulate excess mucous production in the lungs, resulting in the type of asthma triggered by exertion.

## Milk and the immune system

Milk is responsible for more allergies in Britain and the US than any other food.[15] Symptoms may range from stomach pain, diarrhoea, rashes and eczema, migraine, irritable bowel syndrome (IBS), hives and asthma. Intolerance to milk proteins seems most pronounced under the age of three, after which time the child usually *appears* to have outgrown it. However, this may actually be an adaptive mechanism in which the body stops reacting overtly and symptoms go underground. According to the concept of the 'general adaptation syndrome' developed by Hans Seyle, stress has three distinct stages: **alarm**, **adaptation** and, finally, **exhaustion**. For example, you may remember experiencing a heady rush when you tried your first cigarette. Had you continued to smoke, your body would subsequently have moved into adaptation. The same process may be occurring in milk-allergic children. A study quoted by Dr Cordain[16] revealed that 50 per cent of infants with milk allergy went on to develop a range of food allergies before puberty, even though they *appeared* to have recovered from their milk allergy. The **alarm** stage in this case would have been characterised by three years of high reactivity or allergy, followed by the **adaptive** phase marked by an absence of symptoms, later giving way to **exhaustion**, manifesting as multiple allergies. It would be interesting to see whether there exists a correlation between infantile milk allergies and the later development of autoimmune diseases.

Like grains, there is a proven link between milk proteins and autoimmune diseases. One of the most problematic of milk proteins is bovine serum albumin, or 'BSA', which is remarkably similar to the collagen in our joints and to the pancreatic cells that produce insulin. Pasteurisation may be responsible for the increase in autoimmune diseases today. First introduced around 100 years ago to prevent infection, pasteurisation so disfigures the milk proteins that they can trick the immune system into mounting an antibody response which, through the process of molecular mimicry, may then attack the body's own tissues.

As we have already observed, non-organic milk contains high levels of growth hormone and **insulin-like growth factor**, which are associated with cancer and weight gain. Due to excessive milking (yields may be forced up from 500 lb of milk per cow annually to 30,000 lb by drugs) the udders are often chronically infected. The milk is likely to be contaminated with antibiotic residues, contributing to the problem of antibiotic-resistant bacteria. The British Allergy Foundation estimates that 45 per cent of the UK population is allergic to milk. However, this does not take into account intolerances caused by problems metabolising milk or autoimmune diseases.

Although found in all foods, milk contains potentially toxic levels of **lectins**, which are primed to enter the blood stream. You may recall the problems that can ensue when we discussed the wheat lectin WGA, which causes blood cells to clump together. Lectins can also interfere with cell replication and the destruction of old blood cells.

A meta-analysis carried out in 2007 at the Harvard School of Public Health[17] discovered an 80 per cent increased risk of developing Parkinson's disease amongst male dairy drinkers, and although the exact mechanism is not yet understood, this was confirmed by Japanese findings, in which an intake of 10 ounces of dairy per day increased the risk of Parkinson's disease by a staggering 130 per cent. Parkinson's disease is associated with chronic pesticide exposure and failure of detox enzymes that also break down the wheat and milk proteins, gluten and casein. Whether the enzymatic damage is initiated by abnormal food proteins, or whether pesticides render the body unable to metabolise gluten and casein, is not known.

## Cataracts

Vivisectionists routinely induce cataracts in experimental animals by feeding them a high-milk diet. Galactose is one of the sugars found in milk and it accumulates in the lenses of cataract sufferers in the form of galactitol.[18] Dr Cordain states that 42 per cent of people over the age of 52 have cataracts.[19] Needless to say, hunter-gatherers would not have been able to do much in the way of hunting and gathering if they hadn't been able to see.

## Milk and zinc

Despite the claims of the dairy industry, milk actually impedes uptake of vitamins and minerals, with calcium and zinc being most affected. Zinc is needed for the development and health of the brain and nervous system, for blood sugar regulation, immune function, detoxification, joint and skin health, and hormonal balance. Nonetheless, it is estimated that 80 per cent of us are deficient in zinc. Stretch marks give skin its elasticity if zinc levels are low. They are common in pregnancy because of the high demand for zinc by the developing fetus.

In fact, the developing brain needs a lot of zinc and small head circumference in babies correlates with low zinc status in the mother. Labour is triggered by a drop in zinc[20] and maternal zinc deficiency is a major cause of premature deliveries and postnatal depression, as zinc is necessary for making hormones. In children, zinc deficiency is associated with ADHD, behavioural problems, delinquency and anorexia nervosa. Milk contains very little zinc, but what little there is cannot be absorbed due to its high calcium content.

## Is the dairy industry pulling the wool past your eyes?

The development of concentration camps housing sometimes up to 80,000 intensively reared dairy cows servicing the perceived need for milk is an abomination to any civilised society. Implicit in its cheapness and wide availability is the notion that milk is a staple of the human diet. Nothing could be further from the truth as prior to industrialisation very little milk was available. Cows are designed to lactate in response to the birth of a calf, and produce a fairly meagre yield. Calves born to dairy cows have to be fed an alternative formula to free up the udders for humans. This may necessitate the culling of males and the recycling of the females into cash cows. The transformation of grazing cow into factory-farmed milking machine has only been made possible by pharmaceutical drugs and innovations in agricultural technology. The milk that is produced by this system is a hybrid of genetic engineering, hormonal manipulation, antibiotic suppression and greed. Denatured from high-pressure heat treatments, watery and devoid of nutrients but high in chemical residues, it is far removed from the healthy image we have been conditioned to associate with milk.

Modern milk is nothing like the raw, cultured dairy product of 100 years ago. Fermented into yoghurt or cheese as a means of preservation, and undamaged by processes like pasteurisation and homogenisation, raw milk was not associated with allergies and was a rare treat. Note the word 'rare'. For hundreds of years the average cow produced less than a pint a day and this tended to be used to make butter which was stored for the winter. Since 21 lb of milk are needed to make a pound of butter,[21] this left very little for drinking and cheese-making, making milk a precious commodity. By the 1800s the yield had gone up to just under two quarts, or slightly less than two litres, per cow per day, and this increased to nine quarts in the 1960s. Today, thanks to intensive rearing, genetic engineering and routine drugging, dairy cows can now churn out (pun intended) up to 50 quarts per day.

The best feed for cows is green grass in spring, summer and autumn, and silage, hay and root vegetables in the winter. Intensively reared cows, who may never have seen grass let alone eaten it, are fed other foodstuffs instead, producing meat and milk that are completely different in nutritional value, taste and texture. A factory-farmed cow is likely to enjoy a diet that includes soy, cottonseed meal, waste from battery-farmed animals, chicken manure or citrus peel cake which is laced with chemicals that are then passed into the milk.

Grass-fed cows produce milk that is higher in the fat soluble vitamins: A, D, E and K. Today, most milk – even milk labelled 'organic' – may have come from cows that have been kept in confinement all their lives. The advent of agribusiness has made it possible to mass produce oceans of milk and this has led to a dramatic rise over the last few decades in the amount of milk consumed. So, even though milk was part of the post-Paleo diet, it was taken sparingly and was not adulterated as it is today.

## Raw deal

Originally, developed as a means of preservation, the advent of pasteurisation meant that milk could be mass produced for the first time. When milk stepped up into the big business arena, profit rather than health began to determine policy. Originally introduced in 1908, pasteurisation was widely condemned by dieticians and doctors[22] because of its destruction of vitamins and minerals and the denaturing of its proteins. Imagine boiling a strawberry and you might get an idea of how far removed modern milk is from its raw predecessor. Processes such as pasteurisation, skimming off the fat and homogenisation are modern innovations and are extremely destructive processes. Pasteurisation kills beneficial bacteria whilst leaving intact pesticides, herbicides and the organism associated with Johne's disease, with which many intensively reared cows are infected, and which is suspected of causing Crohn's disease in humans. To solve this problem, much commercial milk today is ultra-pasteurised. Ultra-pasteurisation is a violent process that takes milk from a chilled temperature to 125°C in less than two seconds, completely destroying almost all of its nutrients.

Furthermore, the intense heat of pasteurisation alters the structure of milk proteins such as casein and bovine serum albumin, the protein we met earlier in connection with diabetes and rheumatoid arthritis. Casein, which is similar in structure to gluten, is particularly vulnerable to heat damage and an inability to metabolise it is often found in autism, schizophrenia, chronic fatigue syndrome and mental health problems, including eating disorders. Not only does pasteurisation destroy the proteins in milk, but it also destroys the vitamins, renders minerals such as calcium, magnesium, phosphorus and sulphur less absorbable, and damages the enzymes making it even harder to digest.

Prior to pasteurisation, milk had been regarded as a healthy food. There is a link between pasteurised milk and tooth decay, colic in babies, growth problems in children, asthma, hay fever, osteoporosis, arthritis, heart disease and cancer. In fact, calves fed on pasteurised milk die within six weeks.

The fears around tuberculosis from unpasteurised milk have been exaggerated to justify a process designed to maximise profit rather than protect the public from infection. Pasteurisation was introduced as a means of prolonging the shelf-life and enabling those living in urban environments to consume milk that was old. Since pasteurised milk can become putrid, processors must also remove the waste matter by a process of 'centrifugal clarification', which further damages the structure of the milk. However, raw (unpasteurised) milk simply turns into yoghurt when old. Originally introduced to combat TB, infant diarrhoea, undulant fever and other diseases, pasteurisation has morphed modern milk from a food into a poison. Infections amongst cows are caused by poor animal nutrition and dirty production methods and affect those reared in the over-crowded conditions which characterise the modern factory farm. Grazing cows rarely require treatments for infections. Today, modern stainless-steel tanks, milking machines, refrigerated trucks and inspection methods make pasteurisation unnecessary. But, as you shall see, pasteurisation isn't the only way to destroy milk.

## Homogenisation

Homogenisation is a process that breaks down butterfat globules to a tenth of their original size, so they do not rise to the top. This renders the fats useless and prevents the absorption of milk's fat-soluble vitamins. Nevertheless, most milk found in supermarkets today is both pasteurised and homogenised. Drs Kurt Oster and Donald Ross carried out research into the link between the milk protein xanthine oxidase and heart disease. This is the protein found in the artery walls of artherosclerotics. Higher levels of antibodies to milk proteins generally are found in patients with atherosclerosis, increasing in proportion to the amount of *homogenised* milk ingested.

Drs Oster and Ross identified a correlation between death rates from atherosclerosis and degenerative heart disease and homogenised milk. Normal-sized fat molecules would not naturally cross the intestinal barrier, but the homogenisation process forces them through a fine filter at high pressure, which makes them small enough to leach into the body through the gut wall. Furthermore, homogenisation makes fat molecules more resistant to digestion, so they enter the blood stream in an undigested state. It was later discovered that IGF (insulin-like growth factor) could hitch a ride on the backs of these miniaturised fat particles and thus was being piggy-backed into the body by these abnormally small fat particles, providing a further mechanism by which modern milk could disrupt blood sugar regulation.

## Frankenstein farming and milk

Keen to milk milk for all its worth, the dairy industry did not lag behind when it came to genetic engineering. Despite the fact that 95 per cent of farmers initially refused to inject their cows with modified hormones as it made them ill and more prone to mastitis (the cows, not the farmers), pressure from the pharmaceutical industry ensured it caught on nevertheless. However, the labelling of milk as genetically engineered was rejected on the grounds that the 'public wouldn't buy it'. So, today it is impossible to know whether the milk you are consuming does or does not contain genetically engineered hormones.

A naturally occurring cow hormone, 'recombinant bovine growth hormone' (rbGH),[23] was combined with bacteria in the 1990s thus enabling it to be mass produced and then injected into cows. Unfortunately, rbGH substantially increases levels of IGF-1 in milk[24] which is associated with insulin resistance, but is not destroyed by pasteurisation or digestion. Samuel Epstein, MD, Professor of Occupational and Environmental Medicine at the Illinois School of Public Health, went on record as saying that, '...it is highly likely that IGF-1 helps transform normal breast tissue to cancerous cells, and enables malignant human breast cancer cells to invade and spread to distant organs.'

This is understandable since the reason for giving the drug is to stimulate the udders. The fact that it does the same in humans is just an unfortunate side effect. The rise in prostate cancer, which is the male equivalent of breast cancer in that it is associated with excess oestrogen, is likely also to be linked. According to the manufacturer's instructions, rbGH '...increases the risk of mastitis and has been associated with increases in somatic cell counts'. Translated into English, that means infection and pus formation. Unsurprisingly, infections amongst rbGH treated herds increased by 80 per cent necessitating antibiotic treatments. In fact, 80 per cent of the world's antibiotics are given to farm animals, their waste products contaminating the environment and waterways whilst bacteria generally are transforming into resistant superbugs.

## Skimming over the facts

Two popular misconceptions – that fat is fattening and unhealthy and therefore skimmed milk or low-fat foods are good for us – seem to have taken hold in a very short time thanks to the fat phobia generated by the pharmaceutical industry, which is hell bent on getting everyone over 50 on statins. Fat is burned for energy in the body and cannot be stored as fat, *except in the presence of carbohydrate.*[25] When the fat content of a food is reduced by technology it is replaced by carbohydrate, thus making it *more* fattening because it is higher in sugar – a fact that the weight-loss industry has failed to flag up. Any carbohydrate not used for energy is converted to fat and stored in the form of excess weight, either as invisible visceral fat around the organs, as sludge in the liver, or as the all-too-visible flab that many are lugging around today.

We are perfectly able to survive on a diet of fat and protein as our bodies can make carbohydrate when needed. That is why it is possible to suffer from a protein or fat deficiency, but not from a deficiency of carbohydrate. Any foods labelled 'low fat' will inevitably be high in carbohydrate, and the replacement of fat by carbohydrate (sugar) in low-fat foods is the reason they encourage weight gain and reduce energy levels, which is good for the diet industry – but not so good for the would-be slimmer.

The success of the propaganda initiative against fat has seen the fat content of foods, like milk and meat, dropping over the last few decades. Today only 25 per cent of milk sold is full fat which suggests that 75 per cent of the population have fallen for the 'fat is bad' myth and believe that low-fat milk is healthier. The average butterfat content of milk 100 years ago was 4 per cent (or more than 50 per cent of calories),[26] and skimmed milk had not been invented. Now butterfat comprises less than 3 per cent, or less than 35 per cent of calories. Since protein becomes toxic when consumed without fat, the modern trend for low-fat milk and meat not only poses a health problem, but has also resulted in a loss of flavour and texture. Protein and fat are always found together – or at least they were, before man decided he could improve things.

Most consumers are unaware that unless milk contains its full complement of fats its vitamins and minerals cannot be properly absorbed, especially the fat-soluble vitamins, including D and K, both of which are essential for incorporating calcium into bone. You may remember that Dr Weston Price found levels of fat soluble vitamins to be ten times higher in indigenous diets compared to those of the 1930s and '40s. How they would compare with today's is anyone's guess.

Intensively produced milk is watery and lacking in nutrients and would not sustain a calf. It is only by marketing low-fat and skimmed milk as a health food can dairy farmers get shot of the poor-quality, watery milk produced by high-production herds. Furthermore, since butter is produced by removing the fat from milk a market for low-fat milk had to be created to satisfy the demand for butter. Meanwhile the erroneous belief that consuming fat makes you fat made the overweight the ideal target market. With obesity rising to epidemic levels due to the high intake of carbs in the modern diet, there would be no shortage of potential consumers.

## Powdered milk

If you thought skimmed milk was a bad idea, powdered milk is even worse. When milk is powdered (dried), it becomes a source of dangerous oxidised cholesterol, which is neurotoxic (poisonous to the brain). Powdered, skimmed milk is added to 1 per cent and 2 per cent fat milk and to low-fat yoghurts. It is also added to ice-cream and sour cream in the form of mucopolysaccharide slime to camouflage the lack of body and the watery consistency. It is in powdered form that formula milks for babies are produced.

Whilst many of the problems associated with milk are undoubtedly due to industrialised production methods, there is no escaping the fact that milk is primarily a baby food which many are not able to digest after weaning. However, the prevalence of allergies, chronic viral infections and autoimmune diseases today may make undenatured whey or raw milk beneficial additions to the diet for those who can tolerate them, although they may need to be avoided, at least temporarily. Even though raw milk and butter were included in some hunter-gatherer diets, most modern Paleo dieters shun all forms of dairy. However, dairy and grain intolerances were unknown before the Industrial Revolution. Unfortunately, once the body has been triggered by a food, going back to a more natural form of that food, like organic spelt or raw milk, for example, is rarely enough. A period of complete avoidance, combined with natural treatments to boost gut health and immunity, is often required. It is likely that widespread intolerances to wheat and dairy are in part responsible for the popularity of the Paleo diet.

I believe it is healthier to include raw butter (and wild, oily fish) in your diet as Paleo meat was very different from the meat available to us today. Lower in fat generally, and in DHA (see page 11) and CLA (see page 103) in particular, it would be a mistake to rely on modern muscle meat to satisfy your fat requirements. Hunter-gatherers ate the DNA-rich brain, followed by the organs and glands, often wasting the muscle meats because of their comparatively poor nutritional content.

Dr Cordain was correct in writing[27] '…we have been misled by the dairy manufacturer's overhyped advertising and marketing campaigns. It is clear that dairy doesn't prevent bone fractures, and it might contribute to heart disease and cancer...' However, I think the modern version of the Paleo diet needs to be adapted. Pollution substantially increases our need for nutrients. Our immune systems have been changed by a diet high in sugar and by drugs, including steroids, antibiotics and vaccines. The modern digestive system, often chronically constipated and low in digestive juices and beneficial bacteria, would struggle to process an authentic Paleo diet. Incidentally, Dr Cordain recommends eating Paleo 80 per cent of the time and has publicly stated that his preferred source of dietary fat is butter.

## Quick recap

- Milk contains a sugar called lactose.
- Calcium in milk is not readily available, especially if the milk has been pasteurised.
- Acne is linked to sugar and dairy consumption and is not found in indigenous peoples.
- Milk has a destabilising effect on blood sugar.

## Personal health check

Could you be **sensitive to dairy**? Tick any of the following that apply to you or your family:

| | | | |
|---|---|---|---|
| | Sinus congestion | | Hay fever |
| | Asthma | | Eczema |
| | Irritable bowel or tendency to diarrhoea | | Food cravings |
| | Diabetes | | Autoimmune disease |
| | Hormonal problems | | Atherosclerosis |

| | Heart disease | | Stones in gall bladder or kidneys |
|---|---|---|---|
| | Bone spurs | | Osteoporosis |
| | Infantile colic | | Autism, chronic fatigue, learning difficulties, behavioural problems |
| | Acne | | Early or delayed puberty |
| | Weight problems | | Indigestion |

# Chapter 4

# Has beans

## Beans may be just a lot of hot air

Known for their tendency to cause flatulence, beans and other legumes can compete against grains and dairy when it comes to symptoms like indigestion. Legumes include lentils, haricots, kidney and black-eyed and green beans, broad beans and peas. Often assumed to be a healthy alternative to meat, they are much loved by the diet dictocrats. Capable of causing nausea, vomiting, diarrhoea, muscle weakness and inflammation of the heart, unless soaked, boiled or sprouted beans in their raw state are toxic. Dr Cordain recommends that we '…proceed cautiously as we consider the nutritional benefits and liabilities of beans and legumes'.

To test the assumption that beans are a good source of protein for vegetarians, Dr Cordain compared levels in legumes, eggs and meat, and found that meat greatly outstripped legumes. For every 100 kilocalories, turkey and chicken provided 20.1 grams of protein, sea foods 17.9 grams and beef and pork 17.8 grams respectively. Next in line were eggs with 8.1 grams per 1000 kilocalories, whilst legumes came in last with 6.9 grams. This means that legumes contain 66 per cent less protein than white meat and 61 per cent less than red. However, were the figures adjusted to take resistance to digestion into account, the protein values would fall by a further 20 to 25 per cent. The World Health Organisation has devised an index called the 'Protein Digestibility-Corrected Amino Acid Score', or PDCAAS,[1] which shows that beans and pulses are second-rate sources of protein compared with meat and fish. This means that not only do legumes contain significantly less protein than animal foods, but since the human digestive system is not efficient at processing them, what little they do contain is difficult and energy-expensive to extract. Furthermore, like grains, they are awash with anti-nutrients which are toxic to humans and which make them fairly resistant to digestion.

Not a single legume contains all the essential proteins, with cysteine and methionine, two amino acids needed for detoxification, being especially lacking. Vegetarians claim that it is possible to overcome this by combining them with grains, but this would give you a massive carbohydrate hit for a small amount of indigestible protein.

Further research into the nutritional value of pulses gives little cause for optimism. In *The Paleo Answer*, Dr Cordain, who is the only person to have carried out such studies, describes his findings after comparing the mineral levels of legumes, meat, fish and eggs. Although iron tended to be equal or higher, some qualification is needed to put this into context. Iron from non-animal sources is not very useful to humans, with only around 25 per cent being absorbed as it is bound to phytic acid, thus reducing its rating by up to 80 per cent. Iron from animal sources, however, comes in the form of 'haem' iron and, as its name implies, is much more efficient at binding to red blood cells to form haemoglobin.

This is a pattern that is repeated with all the minerals, particularly zinc, with seafoods taking star billing in the zinc ratings. Zinc is essential for sex hormone production and the health of sperm, and it is their high zinc content that has given oysters a reputation for being aphrodisiac. Whilst the zinc levels of legumes were found to be the same as those of white meat at 0.9 grams per 100 kilocalories, they were substantially lower than sea foods, which contain an average of 7.6 grams. The decreased availability of zinc from pulses is unfortunate for vegetarians, whose high intake of carbs increases their demand for insulin, a hormone that is dependent on zinc.

Not only are legumes a poor source of nutrition, they are the outright winners when it comes to anti-nutrients, with levels that would put even grains to shame. The roll call of antinutrients is impressive and includes[2] lectins (which we have already encountered – see page 24), saponins (a soap-like substance that punches holes in the gut wall with the vigour of a machine gun), phytic acid (our old friend with an enduring attraction for minerals – see page 18), polyphenols (which have hormonal effects), protease inhibitors (which switch off protein-digesting enzymes), raffinose oligosaccharides (which cause wind and bloating), cyanogenetic glycosides (which interfere with iodine metabolism, causing goitres and hypothyroidism), and last, but not least, favism glycosides, to which certain genetic groups are highly allergic. Fermenting and sprouting can negate many of the above but does not destroy them completely. Not bad for the humble bean regarded by many, including the government, as a superior food to meat. This mistaken belief is why legumes find themselves in pride of place at the bottom of the infamous food pyramid (see page 9), alongside that other wholesome food – grains. Let's take a look at each of these anti-nutrients in a little more detail.

## Full of beans

### Lectins

All foods contain lectins but those found in vegetables and fruits are quite benign and are usually well tolerated. What makes the lectins from non-Paleo foods like grains, legumes and dairy so toxic is their ability to punch holes in the gut, cross the intestinal barrier and enter the blood stream like looters after a riot. Once in the body they become a law unto themselves, outsmarting the immune system and screwing up the cells. Lectins evolved to protect plants against predators and the way they ensure survival is to release toxins. The fact that many survive digestion intact is due to their ability to cause food poisoning. Kidney beans are the outstanding winners in this category together with other beans from the aptly named *Phaseolus vulgaris* family, to which many pulses belong. These include adukis, black beans, cannellini beans, lima beans, butter beans, haricot beans and pinto beans, all of which are high in a lectin called 'phytohaemagglutinin', or PHA. As its name suggests, this lectin has much in common with our other friend, WGA (the lectin found in wheat) for its talent at gluing red blood cells together. Bean lectins go one stage further, however, by gumming up white blood cells as well. Although the name 'phytohaemagglutannin' might look a bit mind-boggling, it aptly describes what it is: 'phyto' means plant and 'haem' means blood. Translated from Greek into English, 'phyto-haema-gglutannin' simply means 'plant that sticks blood cells together'. Coming in two strains: PHA-L which has a particular affinity for 'leucocytes', a type of white blood cell that is part of the immune system, and PHA-E (the E standing for 'erythrocyte', or red blood cell); it can cause clumping of both.

Not satisfied with silting up the blood, PHA also interferes with the transportation of protein into cells by making their membranes less permeable. Protein is essential for cellular function and reproduction. 'Mitosis' is the biological name for cell division and is the process by which cells divide to produce the next generation of cells that are identical to them. The fact that PHA stimulates mitosis in cells that may also be deficient in protein means that cellular reproduction could get a bit out of hand, and this is what happens in cancer. Animal studies have shown that PHA can disrupt normal cell function and cause disease. It also causes leaky gut, resulting in low-level chronic inflammation in the blood,[3] a precursor to atherosclerosis and cancer. So PHA can make the gut more permeable but the cells less so. Any food that can do this might need to be reclassified as a health hazard!

PHA toxicity is lessened, but not completely neutralised, by cooking. Temperatures of 100 degrees centigrade can reduce PHA to safe levels. 'Safe levels' means levels too low to produce food poisoning but not destroyed completely. However, temperatures less than 100 degrees centigrade, such as those reached by slow cooking, could be even more lethal because cooking beans of the *Phaseolus vulgaris* family at 80 degrees centigrade will increase the toxicity of PHA five-fold.

At the same time, you should be aware that, although they are classified as a legume, green beans are consumed for their pods and at a stage when the bean inside is largely immature. For these reasons they do not present the same problems and are a good source of nutrition and fibre.

## Peanuts

Not really a nut at all but classified as a legume, peanuts have their own special lectin called 'pea-nut-agglutinnin', or PNA. PNA doesn't hang about. It gets into the blood stream within one hour of ingestion. Lentils and peas are the least toxic, with comparatively low levels of lectin, but they too have the ability to damage the gut wall, cause inflammation, impair growth and disrupt immune function[4] in some individuals.

Research over the last 60 years has revealed that the fat in peanuts is highly atherogenic,[5] which means it can cause the formation of plaque along artery walls in experimental animals. Indeed, so successful is it at producing atherosclerosis that it is routinely fed to laboratory rabbits specifically for this purpose. Peanut oil was detected in the blood stream one to four hours after eating a bag of roasted, salted peanuts – in humans that is – and at levels high enough to induce atherosclerotic change in experimental animals.[6] Once in the body, peanut lectins will often bind to the cells that line the artery walls. Peanuts also contain something called an 'aflatoxin', a waste product produced by a fungus called *Aspergillus*, which is highly carcinogenic, or cancer causing.

## Saponins

Saponins have soap-like properties and are found in all legumes. They not only blast holes in the gut wall but they also cause cell membranes to become leaky, and if this occurs in a red blood cell, it can temporarily lose its ability to carry oxygen.[7] Unlike lectins, saponins are unaffected by cooking; however, other methods of preparation, like fermenting or sprouting, destroys some of them. The highest levels of saponins are found in soya beans, which contain 10,600 milligrams per kilograms, followed by TVP ('textured vegetable protein' derived from soy), which contains 4,510 milligrams per kilograms,[8] whereas soy tempeh has only 1,530 milligrams per kilogram, showing the effectiveness of fermentation in decreasing the toxicity of legumes. The next highest, haricot beans, comes in at 3,800, with peanuts containing the lowest level of saponins at 100 milligrams per kilo.

## Polyphenols

Polyphenols are compounds found in plants that protect them from sunlight damage and predators.[9] They come in many forms, some of which are very beneficial. However, two types of polyphenol – tannins and isoflavones – can have adverse effects on health. Similar to phytic acid (see page 18), tannins interfere with protein digestion, bind up minerals and damage the integrity of the gut wall, making it more porous. These three mechanisms for damaging the gut wall would make leaky gut an inevitability on a diet high in pulses. Soy beans boast the highest levels of isoflavones – so high in fact that they are used therapeutically as an alternative to HRT (see chapter 5, page 68).

## Protease inhibitors

The usual suspects, protease inhibitors (see page 43), are rearing their ugly heads again. As their name suggests, they stop protein-digesting enzymes from working. Protein-digesting enzymes are only active in the acidic environment of the stomach. The small intestine, on the other hand, is alkaline and therefore more suited to carbohydrate digestion. However, the arrival of incompletely digested protein from the stomach will force the release of excessive levels of pancreatic enzymes which, over time, can lead to pancreatic enlargement. Spewing protein-digesting enzymes into the small intestine is not without its problems as they can also digest the gut itself, causing our old friend, leaky gut. (This does not occur in the stomach, where there are protective secretions that prevent it from digesting itself.) So although up to 80 per cent of protease inhibitors may be destroyed by cooking, those that do survive are fully equipped to cause digestive mayhem.

## Raffinose oligosaccharides[10]

Raffinose oligosaccharides are made up of three sugars that need to be split into galactose, fructose and glucose by an enzyme called alpha-galactosidase. You don't need to familiarise yourself with sugar digestion but you do need to know that alpha-galactosidase is an enzyme that humans do not have. (Raffinose oligosaccharides are also found in vegetables like sprouts and broccoli but in much smaller quantities so rarely present a problem.) Our lack of alpha-galactosidase makes the raffinose sugars indigestible, necessitating the intervention of fermenting bacteria. This is a case of both good news and bad news. Whilst the bacteria solve the immediate problem of breaking down the sugars, they achieve this by fermenting them into gases such as hydrogen, carbon dioxide and methane which unsurprisingly cause bloating and wind. Moreover, if the gut wall is leaky (*if?!...* *because* the gut wall is leaky), these gases can enter the blood stream causing brain fog and sluggishness.

### Cyanogenetic glycosides[1]

A 'glycoside' is a sugar bound to a non-sugar, and in the case of cyanogenetic glycosides the non-sugar comes in the form of cyanide. Luckily these are largely destroyed by cooking, but those that do survive are broken down to hydrogen cyanide in the gut. If you are fond of Victorian murder mysteries you may have come across cyanide before. Found predominantly in lima beans, hydrogen cyanide is eventually converted into 'thiocyanate', which impairs the uptake of iodine, a mineral essential for thyroid hormone production. Classified as a **goitrogen**, if eaten in large amounts it can cause hypothyroidism so may be best avoided by anyone low in iodine.

### Favism glycosides

Four hundred million people worldwide have a genetic defect in an enzyme called G6PD[12] which breaks down 'favism glycosides', the sugars in broad beans. Associated with increased protection against malaria, this genetic deficit is more common in Middle Eastern, North African and Mediterranean countries. Failure to break down the sugars in broad beans is known as 'favism', and can result in rupture of red blood cells or haemolytic anaemia. The exact mechanisms that cause favism are incompletely understood as not everyone carrying this gene code reacts to broad beans.

## Conclusion

From the lack of enzymes to digest them, their high loading of anti-nutrients and their poor nutritional value, it seems evident that legumes would not constitute the best food choice for humans. Like grains, they are a second-rate source of nutrition whilst being energy expensive. In spite of this, however, governments continue to advocate a low-meat, high-plant food diet for health and to promote legumes as a good source of protein.

### Quick recap

- Legumes contain anti-nutrients, such as phytic acid and enzyme inhibitors.
- The mineral zinc is particularly low in legumes.
- Lectins get into the body through the gut wall.
- Saponins are harmful because they can cause the gut wall to be leaky.

# Chapter 5

# Not soy good for you

In less than a century, soy has gone from being a minor crop mostly used to fix nitrogen in the soil,[1] to being cultivated on an industrial scale and fed to humans. Never eaten without prior fermentation, it transpires that soy was not the great dietary staple of the Asian diet after all. Cheap to produce, and a food manufacturer's dream, soy is now added to many convenience foods, including dairy. Hailed as a 'new miracle food',[2] soy was launched with a fanfare of extravagant health claims, most of which have since turned out to be false.

Having discovered that dairy doesn't agree with you, you may – like many health conscious individuals – have switched to soy believing it to be a good source of protein or a healthy alternative to milk. Indeed, there have been many studies, unfortunately underwritten by the soybean industry, that claim numerous health benefits for soy, many of which have been particularly targeted at the vegetarian population. Unluckily, like the studies on fat, these too are the product of bad science,[3] or what passes for science in this economically driven age. Labelling can be misleading, since soy can hide behind vague names such as 'bouillon', 'lecithin' or 'natural flavour', so you could be consuming it without even realising it. So incriminating is the evidence against soy that it warrants a whole chapter to itself. Let us therefore bypass the hyperbole and look at the evidence.

You may have come across studies boasting lower rates of breast and uterine cancers in Asian women, and lower rates of prostate cancer in the men. Unfortunately, these studies ignore the fact that Asian diets are different in many other ways from those of the West, and also that rates of other cancers such as oesophageal, stomach, pancreatic and thyroid are, in fact, *higher* amongst Asians. Even more surprising is the fact that the Asian diet actually contains so little soy that it would be difficult to extrapolate any conclusions about soy from dietary analysis alone. A study conducted in the 1930s found that soy accounted for as little as 1.5 per cent of calories in the Chinese diet, compared with 65 per cent of calories from pork, so we might reasonably deduce from these studies that eating pork could be protective against hormonal cancers![4] Originally regarded as a fertiliser, *the Chinese didn't consider soy as edible until comparatively recently*.

## Soy, the gender bending bean

Unknown to our Paleolithic ancestors, soy has been linked to many reproductive problems, particularly birth defects, stillbirths and deformities. In fact, so damning was the evidence against soy, that in 1998 the New Zealand Government issued a health warning against the use of soy infant formula, and both Canada and New Zealand have called for it to be banned altogether in formula milks.

We saw in the previous chapter that legumes contain **isoflavones**, a type of polyphenol, which have potent hormonal effects. A recent study found that babies fed soy-based formula had 13,000 to 22,000 times more isoflavones in their blood compared with babies fed milk-based formula.[5] Toxicologist Mike Fitzpatrick, PhD, has identified a correlation between soy consumption and infertility, and researchers at the Institute of Ecology and Evolution at the Russian Academy of Sciences found that hamsters fed GM soy over three generations became infertile.[6] Dr Fitzpatrick also found a connection between dietary intake of soy and cancer, infantile leukaemia and endocrine (hormonal) disruption. Soy has long been known to suppress thyroid function because of its high level of goitrogens, so named – as I described in the previous chapter – because of their thyroid-suppressing effect, which can last for three months. One such goitrogen, **genisten**, was found by the National Centre for Toxicological Research in New Zealand to cause *irreversible* damage to enzymes that make thyroid hormones. Isoflavones too can interfere with thyroid function, sometimes causing cancer and autoimmune thyroid disease.[7] They also have a suppressive effect on the pituitary gland, which helps regulate hormone levels throughout the body. A Japanese study[8] found that as little as 30 grams of soy per day caused a decrease in the release of **thyroid stimulating hormone** from the pituitary, resulting in goitre.

Vegetarian mothers consuming soy have a five-fold greater risk of giving birth to a boy with hypospadias – a birth defect of the penis, otherwise known as 'small willy syndrome'. Soy contains **phytoestrogens** which means oestrogens from plants. So similar are they to our own oestrogens that they can fit on to the cell's hormonal receptors, preventing the body's natural hormones from gaining a foothold. This is why they can have such a profound effect on health, disrupting menstruation, lowering fertility, depressing thyroid function and causing liver problems. The phytoestrogen content of soy is so high that it is estimated that an infant fed on soy-based formula would receive the oestrogenic equivalent of at least five birth control pills per day, so God help him if he's a boy.

Ideally, male foetuses should be exposed to adequate testosterone during the first trimester which is later followed by a surge in testosterone during the first few months of life. Lack of testosterone in early pregnancy has been associated with homosexuality in males, and in monkeys testosterone deficiency during these crucial developmental periods was found to impair learning and cognition.[9] Delayed physical maturation is affecting increasing numbers of boys,[10] and since soy is omnipresent in foods today, its feminising effects on male children are likely to be contributing to this phenomenon. The effects on both sexes of exposure to feminising hormones during pregnancy and early life could potentially hinder thyroid function, and may also increase the risk of infertility and hormonal cancers later in life. In addition, men exposed to dietary soy may also suffer from many feminising traits, including breast enlargement, reduction in facial and bodily hair, loss of libido, impotence and a decrease in sperm count.[11] Eaten by some monks to help suppress their libido, the feminising effects of soy are caused by the **oestrogen mimetics**, genistein and daidzein. Is it possible that soy may also produce the opposite effect in some people, causing a recently recognised condition known as 'sex addiction'? In the book *Trick and Treat*,[12] Barry Groves cites the case of a 44-year-old woman who needed to self-stimulate 15 times a day to relieve pelvic tension, which had started one month after having introduced large amounts of soy into her diet. She was advised to cut out the soy, and lo and behold, all her symptoms, including menstrual problems, were completely resolved within three months.

Considering the adverse hormonal effects soy can engender – no pun intended – it is hardly surprising that it has also been linked to precocious puberty in girls. One per cent of females in the US are showing signs of sexual development, such as pubic hair and breast growth, *before the age of three*, with many others experiencing the early onset of menstruation.[13] Soy may be the smoking gun here since it is more common amongst those of African-American origin, who were the 'lucky' recipients of free soy formula as part of the welfare programme. Early sexual development in girls frequently precedes infertility and breast cancer later in life. Furthermore, GM soy can cause abnormally heavy and longer periods and an increased risk of endometriosis,[14] a disease in which oestrogen-sensitive menstrual tissue migrates to other parts of the body, causing painful internal bleeding at the same time as menstruation.

## GM soy

Found in the form of isolate in a variety of foods including body building powders, protein bars, diet shakes, vegetarian foods, baked goods and even breakfast cereals, soy in the isolate form can amplify its feminising effects, causing erectile dysfunction and decreased libido – which isn't quite the effect the body-builders are after. Soy is made into an isolate by intensive heating and exposure to caustic chemicals, including the carcinogens lysinealine (which further lowers the cysteine content), and nitrosamines.[15] In the US up to 95 per cent of soy is now genetically modified to be resistant to all herbicides with the exception of one called Roundup.[16] This is a deliberate ploy on the part of Monsanto, the producers of both GM soy and Roundup, to trap producers into dependency upon this one pesticide. Roundup is in another league when it comes to toxicity. Its ability to inhibit vital enzyme systems linked to sulphur metabolism have been shown to be fatal in animal experiments. Damage to the digestive and immune systems and the liver and kidneys in humans may be driving many modern health problems, including autism, cardiovascular disease and diabetes. The reason Roundup is so toxic is because it contains **glyphosate**. Glyphosate is a weed-killer that can also disrupt the female reproductive cycle and it is this modified type of soy that is made into isolate. One of the world experts on the effects of Roundup and glyphosate, Dr Stephanie Seneff, warns of a growing epidemic of related health problems.[17]

Pathologist Stanley Ewen says of glyphosate: 'It's an endocrine buster…that interferes with aromatase, which produces oestrogen.' Furthermore, it can increase the risk of miscarriage as it is toxic to the placenta which, in the womb, feeds the developing baby and removes waste products. Even small levels of exposure can cause birth defects. Dr Andres Carrasco of the Embryology Laboratory, Faculty of Medicine in Buenes Aires suggested[18]: '...that abnormally high levels of cancer, birth defects, neonatal mortality, lupus, kidney disease, and skin and respiratory problems in populations near Argentina's soybean fields may be linked to the aerial spraying of Roundup'. May be?!

## Soy and the brain

Soy also appears to be implicated in learning difficulties and behavioural problems whilst consumption of soy in mid-life is linked to cognitive problems, Alzheimer's disease, dementia, and accelerated ageing. A study in the year 2000 on middle-aged tofu eaters revealed brain atrophy and cognitive deficits, correlating with the amount of soy eaten. Eating soy twice or more per week was shown to induce a significant reduction in brain weight. Zinc is an essential mineral for brain and nervous system development during gestation and the first two years of life, and this may be one of the reasons that soy infant formula has been linked to cognitive impairments, although it may also be linked to soy's high aluminium content that is 10 times greater than that of processed milk and a whacking 100 times greater than raw milk.[19] Soy milk lacks cholesterol, a fat essential for brain function, and brains starved of cholesterol can develop dementia, as many statin takers have discovered. In the young, low cholesterol can impede brain development, lowering IQ and causing learning difficulties.

Requirements for vitamin B12, which is also crucial for brain and nervous system function, go up when soy is included in the diet.[20] A deficiency of vitamin B12 is known as **pernicious anaemia**. Only recently has it been realised that B12 from non-animal sources cannot be assimilated, something I wish I had known during my vegan days. Furthermore, drinking grasses like wheat germ and spirulina, which are often consumed regularly by raw foodies and vegetarians in the belief they will provide them with B12, can actually induce B12 deficiency. This is because B12 from plants is in the 'analogue' form, which means it is similar to but not the same as B12 derived from animal sources. This makes it useless to humans because the analogue form blocks uptake of the real vitamin in the same way that phytoestrogens block the uptake of natural oestrogens. Moreover, grasses spirulina and wheatgrass juices are nothing more than liquid cereals with the fibre removed. That would pack a mighty punch of anti-nutrients and allergens. In fact, spirulina is sometimes taken *because* of its high phytic acid levels to remove toxic metals, but since toxins are stored deep within the body it is more likely to pull the minerals out first. Green juices are also high in oxalates which, unless combined with sodium and potassium and converted into harmless salts, can form oxalic acid in the body, causing muscle pain and increasing the risk of stone formation.

In 1980,[21] experimenters demonstrated that young rats fed milk containing soy oil incorporated the oil directly into their brain cells, and had structurally abnormal brain cells as a result. Zinc helps protect the brain against heavy-metal toxicity, so if in short supply, toxic metals such as aluminium, lead and mercury are taken up instead. Furthermore, since the blood-brain barrier becomes porous after eating sugar, it is likely that many children today may be at greater risk of learning difficulties and behavioural problems due to the combined effects of environmental exposure and a diet low in zinc but high in sugar. We have already seen that legumes have many mechanisms that cause leakiness of the intestinal wall. It seems reasonable to surmise that, once in the blood stream, the anti-nutrients that damage the gut wall may also increase permeability of the blood-brain barrier, making it easier for toxins to gain access.

## Anti-nutrients and the processing of soy

Like other legumes, soy too contains protease inhibitors that prevent protein digesting enzymes from working and which in animal studies have been found to cause pancreatic enlargement and cancer. Some manufacturers use heat treatments to remove the anti-nutrients from soy, but the high temperatures required to be effective also damage the proteins in the same way that pasteurisation denatures the proteins in milk. It's a lose-lose situation in which soy protein is either prevented from being digested and absorbed because of its anti-nutrient content, or its proteins are rendered useless by heat treatments.

In common with other pulses, soy is low in a protein called cysteine, which is essential for the metabolism of the other proteins present in the soy.[22] Without cysteine, any soy proteins that may have survived processing cannot be metabolised. Soy is high in polyunsaturated vegetable oil that would become rancid when undergoing heat treatment, turning the fat into free radicals.

Claims that soy prevents osteoporosis cannot be substantiated since soy actively blocks assimilation of calcium and vitamin D, a vitamin needed to get calcium into bone. As we saw in the last chapter, soy contains one of the highest phytic acid levels known and in a form that is in part resistant to fermentation. Phytic acid causes loss of all minerals, but it is the zinc in soy that appears to be particularly vulnerable.

Traditionally soy would have been fermented and eaten in the form of tofu, miso or soy sauce, which is not to be confused with the mass produced, unfermented sugar and MSG-laden (see page 121) liquid that passes for soy sauce today. The advantage of fermentation is that it helps reduce the anti-nutrient levels although it does not completely destroy phytic acid. Unfortunately, modern production of soy products doesn't always use the more time-consuming fermentation method but precipitates the beans instead. Precipitation is the addition of an acid to extract the proteins from the beans in order to make soymeal. Unluckily, precipitation concentrates rather than destroys the enzyme inhibitors, and most commercially produced soya milks are a by-product of this process.

The health claims made for soy apply only to fermented soy, a fact that has not been made clear by its proponents. Even so, fermentation does not neutralise all the anti-nutrients, and since soy is a nutritionally disappointing food with powerful hormonal effects, it probably has no place in a healthy diet.

## Quick recap

- The thyroid gland is vulnerable to the effects of soy.
- The toxic metal aluminium is found in soy.
- Eating soy increases the need for vitamin B12.
- Lysine and methionine are low in soy.

# Chapter 6

# Pseud's corner

In their search for a grain substitute, many turn to alternatives like amarynth and quinoa as they are not technically classified as grains. However, the distinction is more linguistic than scientific. Grains are defined as the seeds of grasses belonging to the Poaceae family.[1] 'A rose by any other name is still a rose,' as Juliet said to Romeo, and this is why seeds such as chia, buckwheat, quinoa and amarynth are almost identical to cereals both in what they contain and how they behave in the body.

Dr Cordain talks of the 'food foraging theory', which has been used by anthropologists to evaluate energy expenditure versus calorific return when studying hunter-gatherer diets.[2] In other words, how much 'bang for your buck' do you get from different foods? Large animals come top of the list, followed by small animals, birds and fish, with cereals coming in last, immediately below nuts and seeds. This means that a nut-, seed- and grain-based diet requires the most preparation and is therefore high in energy and time expenditure but delivers the lowest nutritional return. There is evidence that some hunter-gatherers ate nuts and seeds, but only if their preferred food (meat) was not available, a fact that was confirmed by a study in 2000 of 229 hunter-gatherer diets.[3] Furthermore, since seeds are only available for a few months or weeks per year, their contribution to Paleo nutrition would have been minimal. Compare this to the modern diet in which grass seeds have graduated to prime position, making grains our most commonly eaten food.

Plants don't produce seeds as some sort of philanthropic sacrifice to feed other species. As Dr Cordain points out,[4] were they to do so they would rapidly become extinct. Plants produce seeds as a means of procreation and have therefore evolved a number of strategies to ensure their survival if eaten by predators. Anti-nutrients are a popular method of protection, as we have already seen. They may alternatively house the seed in a hard shell – otherwise known as a nut, or surround it by a soft fruit such as a peach or plum, or they may grow thorns. Fruits that contain stones tend to be high in polysaccharides, a type of sugar that people with irritable bowel syndrome often find difficult to digest and absorb.

Amarynth, quinoa, buckwheat and some other seeds are known as 'pseudo grains', getting off on a technicality since the only difference between them and a cereal is the family to which they belong. Like grains, they have a high loading of anti-nutrients and substandard nutritional content. However, occasional consumption would mimic the way they would have been eaten in Stone Age times. The problem today[5] is that foods are available all year round. Seasonal availability and changes in location meant that foods would traditionally have been eaten on a rotational basis. Today the same foods may be eaten daily, and in quantities that could expose us to levels of anti-nutrients sufficient to induce low-level, chronic inflammation and increase our susceptibility to allergies and autoimmune disease. Part of the reason for the increase in reactions to foods is simply the frequency with which they are eaten. Rotating foods every four days after a period of abstinence can enable a previously allergic person to safely reintroduce a trigger food.

## Chia seeds

Touted by raw foodies as a nutritious and healthy food, chia seeds are the new kids on the block as far as Europeans are concerned, but they have been eaten for thousands of years in South America, where they are sometimes ground into a flour[6] and baked. Although at first glance their nutritional values look impressive, they plummet when the anti-nutrient effects are factored in, especially since they boast one of the highest phytic acid levels known. Furthermore, a food that contains such a high loading of phytic acid could potentially bind up other minerals eaten at the same meal. High in carbohydrate and polyunsaturated fat, they are not the best choice for anyone wishing to lose weight. Chia seeds come in a mucilaginous gel[7] that forms a barrier along the gut wall, preventing nutrient absorption.

## Amaranth

A pseudo grain that is becoming increasingly popular in response to the demand for gluten-free substitutes for flour and cereals, amaranth contains three groups of anti-nutrients[8]: protease inhibitors, saponins and a lectin called 'ACA', or *Amaranthus caudatus*, which has been found to promote cancer cell growth in the intestines. Notable for its high saponin content of 790 milligrams per kilogram, amaranth could also be problematic for people with autism, chronic fatigue syndrome, fibromyalgia and related problems due to its high level of oxalic acid. If oxalic acid ends up in the muscles it can cause stiffness and pain, and if it teams up with bio-unavailable calcium it may form stones in the liver, gall bladder or kidneys.[9]

## Quinoa

Also from South America, quinoa too has impressive levels of anti-nutrients, including saponins, protease inhibitors, phytic acid and tannins. Even higher in saponins than amaranth with a phenomenal 5,000 milligrams per kilogram, quinoa has been shown to cause leaky gut in experimental animals.[10]

## Buckwheat

There has been very little research into buckwheat, but what is known is that, in common with other pseudo grains, it contains high concentrations of protease inhibitors, which switch off protein digestion. In a small minority of people, buckwheat can cause a life-threatening allergic reaction. It also contains something currently unidentified which can react with sunlight and cause a skin reaction.[11]

## Going nuts

Nuts are defined as a 'seed contained within a hard shell' and therefore have many of the disadvantages of seeds and cereals, and, like seeds, would have been eaten infrequently. Prior soaking is often recommended to help remove the anti-nutrients and to make them more digestible, To avoid the sogginess the nuts are then placed in a dehydrator or cool oven, but this requires a little preplanning. Today, nuts are becoming increasingly associated with allergies, although in many cases it is peanuts that are the problem. (As I explained in the previous chapter, peanuts are actually a legume and not a true nut.) The reason for this is thought to be early exposure to peanut oils in nappy-rash creams, as babies lack the enzymes to break them down.

Whilst nuts do not contain saponins, they are high in polyunsaturated fats and carbohydrates and contain anti-nutrients, like protease inhibitors and lectins. Table 1 shows the levels of phytic acid and polyunsaturated fats in some of the most widely eaten nuts. Like peanuts, cashews aren't nuts either but are more accurately classified as a legume. However, I have included them in the list.

**Table 1:** Problem ingredients in nuts

| Nut | Phytic acid in milligrams (mg) per 100 grams | Polyunsaturated fat in grams (g) per 100 grams |
|---|---|---|
| Almonds | 1,280 | 12.1 |
| Cashews | 1,866 | 7.8 |
| Chestnuts | 47 | 0.09 |
| Hazelnuts | 1,620 | 7.9 |
| Macadamia | Very low | 1.5 |
| Walnuts | 760 | 47.2 |

## Veg out

We cannot leave 'Pseud's corner' without mentioning the humble potato, a member of the nightshade, or *solanacea*, family which also includes tomatoes, peppers, aubergine, goji berries and tobacco. Vegetables of the nightshade family were toxic in their wild form and would not have been part of the Stone Age diet. They can worsen arthritis, causing pain and inflammation in affected joints. Potatoes are not great for carb cravers either as they carry the highest **glycaemic loading** of all the root vegetables. Defined as a member of the tuber family,[12] they too contain anti-nutrients. 'Glycaemic load', which was devised in 1997, is a more accurate method of determining the effect of a food on blood sugar than the 'Glycaemic index'. It is easily calculated by multiplying the glycaemic index of a given food by the amount of carbohydrate in a standard portion.[13] Some foods that are high on the glycaemic index are found to have a low glycaemic loading, which means they will not spike the blood sugar. A glycaemic index of 55 or over is considered a high reading.

**Table 2:** Table comparing the glycaemic index of root vegetables with the glycaemic load per 100 grams

| Vegetable | Glycaemic index | Glycaemic load |
|---|---|---|
| Potato, baked | 85 | 21.5 |
| Sweet potato, baked | 61 | 14.8 |
| Beetroot | 64 | 6.4 |
| Carrots | 47 | 4.9 |
| Swede | 71 | 3.4 |
| Turnip | 1-2 | 1-2 |
| Yam | 37 | 10.2 |

Dr Cordain recommends a maximum of 10 GL at one meal for anyone wishing to lose weight or who suffers from blood sugar problems.[14] Athletes, and those engaged in strenuous exercise, have a higher requirement for carbohydrates. Vegetables have the advantage of being alkalising and do not leach calcium from the bones or amino acids from the muscles, making root vegetables a preferable source of energy to grains.

Potatoes contain two saponins called 'glycoalkaloids',[15] which protect them from being attacked by insects, with the highest concentrations being found in the skins which contain between 567 and 1,450 milligrams per kilogram, compared with boiled, peeled potatoes which contain only 27 to 42 milligrams per kilo. One glycoalkaloid, solanine, can cause nausea and gut irritation, headache and neurological symptoms including poor memory and drowsiness. Potatoes that are green or which have sprouted are high in solanine, which is also thought to have teratrogenic effects on developing foetuses. Solanine blocks the actions of an enzyme called 'acetyl cholinesterase' that breaks down acetylcholine, a brain chemical necessary for memory and motor skills, which is low in patients with Alzheimer's disease. Studies on chick embryos found an association between solanine exposure and neural tube defects.

Saponins exert their destructive effects by dissolving cell membranes. Unfortunately, if they permeate the gut wall and get into the blood stream they can dissolve the membranes around red blood cells. Linked to Crohn's disease and ulcerative colitis, potato saponins can also make the gut more leaky.

Some doctors have expressed concern about the potential toxicity of potatoes and questioned whether they would be sanctioned as a food, were they to be introduced today. There is a suspicion that low-level chronic toxicity from the regular consumption of potatoes may be more prevalent than has been realised.[16] Dr Cordain believes they could cause a chronically leaky gut which can be the precursor to inflammation and autoimmune disease. Two studies quoted by Dr Cordain have shown that levels of an antibody called IL6 (interleukin 6) are raised in response to a diet high in potatoes.[17]

Little is known about the effects of potato lectins, although they are known to bind to body tissues and irritate the immune system. Potatoes contain an average of 65 milligrams of lectins per kilogram.[18] Other root vegetables, like beetroot, turnips and so on, do not contain lectins and can therefore be enjoyed as part of a healthy diet.

How potatoes are cooked can also influence their potential for harm. If fried they are likely to contain a neurotoxin called 'acrylamide', or ACR, which is also found in cigarette smoke.[19] ACR is formed when carbohydrates are exposed to high temperatures, with levels increasing the hotter the fat, so deep-fried chips should definitely be off the menu. Although the amount eaten at each sitting may be small, the accumulative effect of a diet high in 'fries' could have a potentially damaging effect, which is worrying when you consider that this is how many children eat potatoes and for some, potatoes may be their only vegetable. Their small body size makes them more vulnerable to the toxic effects of ACR compared with adults, and up to 50 per cent has been found to cross the placenta or get into breast milk. ACR can cause nerve damage, muscle weakness and cancer, and animal studies have shown it to cause foetal abnormalities. Researchers have requested controls over ACR in baby foods, which are subjected to extremely high temperatures during manufacture in order to sterilise them.

Dr Cordain says in *The Paleo Answer*,[20] 'Potatoes should stay underground'.

## Quick recap

- Pseudo grains are classified under a different species but have similar effects in the body.
- Potatoes are different from other root vegetables because they contain saponins which can blow holes in the gut wall, they are highest on the glycaemic index and they inhibit the action of the enzyme acetyl cholinesterase.
- Chia seeds are highest in phytic acid.

# Chapter 7

# Saturated fat – your new best friend

No food has been more misrepresented and maligned than fat. The misguided demand for low-fat foods is a tribute to the ingenuity of the food and chemical industry, but it has had a devastating impact on health. In spite of the fact that saturated animal fat has been our main source of energy since we started walking on two legs – and probably before that – fat has been transformed from a healthy to an unhealthy food in a remarkably short time.

The denigration of fat was initiated by a report published in 1929 by the now infamous Ancel Keys, who jumped to conclusions about the link between fatty foods and health due to his observation that the wealthy and sick in America tended to eat a rich diet. He then looked for epidemiological evidence for his theory. Unfortunately, Keys was selective with his data, only including countries that supported his belief and excluding any that contradicted it, a methodology that was way ahead of its time. As the financial implications of the condemnation of fats were immediately obvious to the chemical, drug and food industries, 'fat is bad' became the new dogma, and has been gaining momentum ever since – not least because it is fed to medical students.

## The lipid hypothesis

Keys's theory became known as the 'lipid hypothesis'. It proposes a relationship between the amount of saturated fat and cholesterol in the diet and the incidence of coronary heart disease. Despite much contradictory research and a dearth of scientific evidence in support of his ideas, the lipid hypothesis was quickly embraced by medical orthodoxy and received far more publicity than could be matched by proponents of traditional foods.

Low-fat diets have repeatedly been shown to be unhealthy. They cause fatigue, impaired cognition, depression, weight gain, blood sugar imbalances, dementia and mineral deficiencies. Nathan Pritikin,[1] a low-fat advocate of the early 1980s, gained media attention for his diet and exercise programme, a regimen that unfortunately led to leukaemia and subsequent suicide when he failed to cure himself.

There is one study often quoted in support of the lipid hypothesis. The effect of a high-cholesterol diet on rabbits was studied by Russian researchers in the early part of the 20th century. The choice of rabbits, who eat a low-fat vegetarian diet of hay and grass and who are have no means of processing cholesterol, was surprising to say the least. Even more damning, however, was the recent discovery that said rabbits were fed a mix of cholesterol *and* polyunsaturated fats, making it impossible to support the study's conclusion that cholesterol causes atherosclerosis.

## Fat in the Stone Age diet

In the stampede to incriminate fat, no one seems to have stopped to ask why a food that has been a major part of the human diet for millions of years should suddenly have become bad for us. Traditional diets the world over are high in saturated fat and cholesterol, fats that account for over 50 per cent of the calories in mother's milk. Babies and children need a good intake of both these fats for growth and development, and failure to thrive is a known consequence of saturated fat deficiency. Both cholesterol and saturated fat are especially important for the developing brain and a deficiency of either can lead to learning difficulties, dyslexia and dyspraxia. Whilst saturated fat in particular, and fat generally, has been scapegoated for all the ills of the modern diet, more obvious contenders – like technological intervention, chemical additives and genetic engineering – have conveniently been overlooked.

## Does it matter if a fat is saturated or poly-unsaturated?

The last few decades have seen enormous changes in the way we eat and the replacement of saturated fats by vegetable oils is a cause for concern. Vegetable oils such as sunflower and safflower are generally polyunsaturated and are vulnerable to rancidity (oxidation). This occurs when they are exposed to heat, including the heat of the body or from cooking, and it is the reason they are associated with numerous health problems. Some researchers, most notably Ray Peat PhD, a biochemist who has been studying fats since 1968, question their essentiality and recommends avoiding them altogether.

The most important thing you need to know about fat is how structurally stable it is. Structural stability enables fats to maintain their shape even when heated. Unstable fats, on the other hand, are unable to do this and become rancid, producing free radicals. Free radicals are atoms with unpaired electrons. Like warriors on the rampage, free radicals attack cell membranes, and once they have gained entry into the cells they damage the genetic coding – DNA and RNA – and trigger tissue mutations. From wrinkles to cancer, free radicals are the health equivalent of weapons of mass destruction.

Saturated fats are held together with strong hydrogen bonds and this gives them stability. The fat is said to be *saturated* with hydrogen and this causes them to remain solid at room temperature. Examples include butter, meat, fish, eggs and goose fat and tropical oils such as coconut and palm – the type of fat that was prevalent in the ancestral diet.

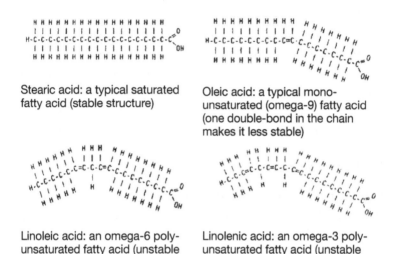

Stearic acid: a typical saturated fatty acid (stable structure)

Oleic acid: a typical mono-unsaturated (omega-9) fatty acid (one double-bond in the chain makes it less stable)

Linoleic acid: an omega-6 poly-unsaturated fatty acid (unstable structure)

Linolenic acid: an omega-3 poly-unsaturated fatty acid (unstable structure)

**Figure 3:** The structures of different fats determines their stability

As you can see, poly-unsaturated fats, or 'PUFAs', have fewer hydrogen bonds, which makes them less stable and causes them to be liquid at room temperature. PUFAs, which include the omega-3 and omega-6 fats, have multiple double bonds. (They are named omega '6' and '3' according to the position of the first double bond). When heated they form free radicals, which makes them unsuitable for cooking. Many societies around the world cured rather than cooked fish as a method of preservation and to protect the oils, and there is a long tradition of this in Scandinavia. Cold smoking was also used, but both curing and cold smoking have become less popular since the invention of refrigeration. Meat fat, which is predominantly saturated, is stable when heated so does not pose the same problems as PUFAs. For example, bone marrow contains only trace levels of omega-3 and omega-6 so would not be damaged by cooking. Omega-6 PUFAs include sunflower, borage and safflower, and walnut and fish oils are omega-3s. The majority of nuts and seeds are high in omega-6.

'Mono-unsaturates', so-named because they only have one double bond, are not as volatile as PUFAs but not as stable as the saturates. They have a kink in their structure, which makes them bend but they are still safe for cooking, providing the temperatures are not too high. Mono-unsaturated fats, of which olive oil is an example, also remain liquid at room temperature.

## PUFAs and health

Only eaten in small amounts by our Paleo ancestors, over the last 50 or so years PUFAs have come to dominate our fat intake. This is a period which has witnessed a rise in degenerative diseases of over 350 per cent. Whilst other factors are undoubtedly involved, the increase in free radicals from dietary PUFAs cannot be ignored. Grass-fed meats contain a minimal amount of fat in the polyunsaturated form, with saturated fat predominating. It is known that saturated fat has an antioxidant effect which neutralises free radicals. The problem today is that saturated fats in the modern diet have been replaced by PUFAs, and in amounts that would never have been found in traditional diets.

PUFAs cause tissue destruction and accumulate in cell membranes, and their proponents claim they are essential for maintaining 'membrane fluidity'.[2] However, according to Peat, polyunsaturated fats and their breakdown products actually *interfere* with 'enzymes and transport proteins and this accounts for many of their toxic effects, so they definitely don't just harmlessly form 'membranes'.[3] On the contrary, Peat regards membrane *fluidity* to be membrane *weakness*. This is a view shared by Dr Mary Enig, an expert in fat nutrition at the Weston Price Organisation.

Many studies have demonstrated a link between PUFAs and cancer, a disease characterised by elevated levels of free radicals. Free radicals (atoms with unpaired electrons) are produced from rancid fats and wreak havoc throughout the body. Like a thief in the night they steal electrons from neighbouring atoms, creating a chain reaction of tissue destruction, and are always found in chronic diseases and inflammation.

PUFAs also slow the metabolic rate which is why they are used by farmers to fatten cattle, and lower the blood sugar. Peat has identified three ways in which they do this:[4]

- by damaging the mitochondria, causing fuel to be burned without useful effect;
- inhibiting energy producing enzymes (both directly and through their anti-thyroid effects) resulting in reduced energy output;
- and by promoting weight gain as they stimulate the conversion of carbohydrate to fat.

## Fat and heart disease

Cardiovascular disease went from being virtually unknown in 1920s' America to becoming the leading cause of death by the 1950s and beyond, a period in which animal fat consumption had been steadily declining. Butter consumption has dropped from 18 pounds per person per year to 4 pounds, whilst the intake of vegetable oils has shot up by around 400 per cent, and refined foods and sugar by 60 per cent. Heart disease now accounts for at least 40 per cent of all deaths in the US and kills 200 people in the UK every day.

A study of British men published in *The Lancet* in 1983 revealed that swopping saturated fat and cholesterol for vegetable oils like margarine resulted in a 100 per cent increase in mortality compared with controls who ate animal fats and smoked. Inexplicably, the author of the study concluded by recommending a reduction in saturated fat intake.[5] The heart surgeon, Michael DeBakey, was unable to find a link between hardening of the arteries and cholesterol levels, and the often cited Framlingham Heart Study, which followed the health of 6,000 men over a 40-year period, found the same. The director of the study said: '...the more saturated fat one ate, the more cholesterol one ate, the more calories one ate, the lower the person's serum cholesterol... we found that the people who ate the most cholesterol, ate the most saturated fat, ate the most calories, weighed the least and were the most physically active.'[6]

Dr Mercola, a well-known champion of alternative medicine and osteopathic doctor, wrote in a 2013 e-newsletter:[7] 'A recent article in the *British Medical Journal*...throws conventional dietary advice on its ear...' 'The myth that vegetable oils (rich in omega-6 fats) are healthier for you than saturated animal fats has been a tough one to dismantle. But the truth cannot be quenched.'

He then goes on to quote from the article: 'Dietary advice about fats and the risk of heart disease is called into question on *bmj.com* today as a clinical trial shows that replacing saturated animal fats with omega-6 polyunsaturated vegetable fats is linked to an *increased* risk of death among patients with heart disease.'

The *British Medical Journal* article was based on a three-year analysis of nearly 500 men aged between 30 and 59, who had recently suffered 'a coronary event'. They were divided into two groups, one of which was placed on a diet high in omega-6s whilst the control group made no changes to their diet. It was found that the risk of dying from heart disease increased by 17 per cent in those in the omega-6 group compared with an 11 per cent in controls, with the omega-6 group showing a higher risk of overall mortality.

Unfortunately, in spite of having been published in the *BMJ*, this research has had no impact on the numbers of statins prescribed, which increases year by year. Statins are drugs prescribed to lower cholesterol based on the erroneous associations between elevated cholesterol and heart disease.

## PUFAs and energy

The reason why those on vegetable oils were less physically active can be explained by the effects of PUFAs on cellular energy production. Inside every cell are little powerhouses called **mitochondria**. They are the furnaces that keep your body working by generating energy. Cells depend upon a good output of energy in order to function. Unfortunately, many people today are not firing on all cylinders. Always found in degenerative diseases and fatigue disorders, mitochondrial damage is commonplace and is due to numerous factors including pollution, stress and the effects of some drugs. Peat believes the high intake of PUFAs in the modern diet to be a significant factor.* Rancid PUFAs not only damage the mitochondria but also suppress the enzyme that repairs them. Jane Collis, an independent researcher, said in the *British Medical Journal* (Rapid Response 12 February 2013): 'Polyunsaturated oils are unstable and very quickly become rancid. Oxidized fatty acids are dangerous to our health.'

PUFAs can lower the metabolic rate in other ways too. Cells make energy in response to stimulation from thyroid hormones, but the more unsaturated the fat, the more it suppresses the action of thyroid hormone.

Peat claims: 'All of these oils, even if they're organic, cold-pressed, unprocessed, bottled in glass, and stored away from heat and light, are damaging. These oils have no shelf life at all, they go rancid within days unless refrigerated, and when they're warmed to body temperature, they disintegrate even faster. Once ingested, they bind with cells and interfere with every chemical reaction in the body. The results are hormone imbalances, inflammation and all kinds of illness'.

---

* Mitochondrial damage has many causes.

Whilst Peat is undoubtedly correct in highlighting the potential for rancidity and metabolic inhibition from extracted oils, he may be incorrect in recommending avoidance of naturally occurring PUFAs since, with the exception of most nuts and seeds, they are usually found with saturates. The ill-effects of PUFAs identified by Peat and other researchers are undoubtedly exacerbated by an imbalanced ratio of omega-6 over omega-3 and the lack of saturated fat and cholesterol in the modern diet.

## Head start

The human brain is high in fat, and in 1978 a study on pregnant mice demonstrated superior brain development in the offspring of mothers fed coconut oil compared with those fed PUFAs. The less stable PUFAs are more than likely to cause free radical damage in the fat-rich brain, something known to occur during seizures. They may also contribute to thrombosis and strokes as they interfere with an enzyme involved in the breakdown of clots. Free-radical damage is also involved in the nerve cell degeneration of Alzheimer's disease, against which cholesterol has a protective effect.[8]

In addition to saturated fat and cholesterol, the omega-3 fat, DHA, appears to have been of particular importance in the evolution of the human brain and is responsible for a dramatic increase in brain size. DHA is found in oily fish and fatty, grass-fed meat.

## Fat facts and fantasies

All of the above flies in the face of much modern health dogma, which warns against eating saturated fat and red meat, and promotes PUFAs as both essential and healthy. Since WWII vegetable oils have been cost effective to extract and once the demand for them dried up as the military had less need of them, a new market had to be found. Butter from grass-fed cows, full-fat milk and coconut oil are relatively expensive to produce and with a much reduced profit margin, are less attractive to manufacturers. This is how industrial oils have been introduced into the human diet.

## Commercially produced oils

Industrially produced oils, like soy, corn and canola, have been introduced into the diet with disastrous consequences. Canola, an unnatural and toxic hybrid made from rapeseed, is so ubiquitous in the modern diet that it deserves special attention. A known toxin which is added to many convenience foods, such as mayonnaises and coleslaws, rapeseed oil is two-thirds erucic acid, which can cause lesions in the heart known as 'Keshan's disease'. For this reason it is used by vivisectors to induce heart damage in experimental animals. After the Canadian military stopped using rapeseed oil in machinery, a selectively bred mutant, canola, was developed in 1978 which contained 60 per cent mono-unsaturated and up to 35 per cent polyunsaturated fat. There is actually no such plant as canola – the name comes from 'Canada Oil Low Acid' – CAN-O-L-A. Along with other industrially produced oils, canola is associated with heart disease and cancer. It is rumoured that the producers paid $50 million to obtain 'GRAS status'. GRAS means 'Generally Regarded As Safe', but this assumption cannot be substantiated as canola was developed from rapeseed that had been banned due to its toxic effects. Things got even worse in 1995 when genetic engineering added three different strains of bacterial DNA to ensure its dependence upon a pesticide called Roundup, with the result that now 82 per cent of all canola oil is contaminated with this pesticide.

Commercially produced PUFAs become oxidised during production during which they are subjected to intense heat, pressure and chemicals including hexane (the petroleum solvent), which is known to damage nerves. Caustic refining, de-gumming (don't ask), bleaching and deodorising are the processes that oils undergo before being bottled. Any omega-3 fats in the oil get transformed into what are called 'trans-fats' and Mary Enig has found levels to be as high as 4.6 per cent. Trans-fats are lipids that do not exist in nature and are created by hydrogenising (adding hydrogen) to liquid fats to make them solid at room temperature. They are often found in processed foods, 'spreads' and margarines.

One of the reasons canola is so detrimental to health is that it causes vitamin E levels to drop rapidly. Vitamin E is important in protecting against lipid peroxidation, the term used to describe the transformation of fats to free radicals. Canola would therefore increase the need for this vitamin whilst simultaneously stripping it from the body. Studies in 1996 and 1997 found canola oil to have been lethal when fed to animals, and as it impedes growth it is not allowed to be added to infant formulas.

## How essential are the essential fats?

'Essential' fatty acids are the omega-3 and omega-6 fats known as PUFAs or poly-unsaturates. They have recently been promoted by health professionals as 'essential' and healthier than saturated fat. However, Peat cites a study in which animals deprived of 'essential fatty acids' demonstrated remarkable properties. 'They consumed oxygen and calories at a very high rate...their mitochondria were unusually tough and stable ...they were very hard to kill by trauma and a wide variety of toxins that easily provoked lethal shock in animals on the usual diet'.[9]

In the 1960s doctors discovered that PUFAs increase graft survival in transplant patients due to their suppressive effect on the immune system.[10] It appears that doctors may be ahead of alternative practitioners in this regard, as they routinely give PUFAs intravenously following organ transplantation *with the specific intention of inhibiting immune function!*

Peat believes PUFAs probably bind to all proteins, disrupting some of them. Their affinity for proteolytic (protein-digesting) and respiration-related (energy producing) enzymes is due to their slightly more water-soluble property compared with fully saturated fats, giving them a greater tendency to concentrate in the cell membranes. So, whilst it is true that the liquid polyunsaturated oils, such as those found in nuts and seeds, do increase 'membrane fluidity', it is now clear that in at least some of those cases the 'fluidity' corresponds to the chaos of a damaged cell protein structure.[11] Furthermore, it has been known for some time that PUFA-induced free-radical damage to red blood cells weakens their structure, making them about as stable as a blancmange and causing them to be prematurely destroyed.[12] It is feasible that other cells would be affected in the same way.

Oxygen is needed for the production of energy, but it is a highly reactive gas. It is therefore hard to believe that in the cells such dangerous fats would find themselves in close proximity to a volatile element like oxygen. It would be like putting oil next to a fire. Saturates, however, are non-reactive with oxygen and not only convey an antioxidant effect but provide efficient fuel for energy.

Whilst saturates have been rebranded as bad, the importance of polyunsaturates, or PUFAs, seems to have been overstated. PUFAs, which are all the rage in nutrition circles, have been elevated to such a level that many health benefits have been attributed to them. Indeed, there is now a thriving industry producing supplements such as evening primrose and fish oil. Cheap to manufacture, PUFAs now account for 30 per cent of the modern diet in spite of the fact that they only contributed a meagre 4 per cent of calories to the ancestral diet, with saturated fat contributing up to 65 per cent and more in the case of the Inuit and Masai.

The most well known of the PUFAs are omega-6 and omega-3.

PUFAs in properly reared, grass-fed meat have a balanced ratio of 1:1 omega-6 to omega-3. However, since the Industrial Revolution there has been a steady increase in the ratio of 6 to 3, with estimates ranging from 10–20:1 today. Not only has omega-6 increased in the modern diet, but omega-3 has gone down as levels in vegetables, eggs, fish and meat have been reduced by industrial food production practices. Free range, organic hens feeding on insects and plants produce eggs with omega-3 fats whereas artificially fed hens produce eggs with up to 19 times more omega-6.

Unless omega-6 is kept in balance with omega-3 it can disrupt the function of chemical messengers called prostaglandins. Prostaglandins mediate muscle contraction and regulate inflammation via a number of pathways. A predominance of omega-6 fats in the diet can result in inflammation, the formation of blood clots, high blood pressure, digestive distress, depressed immunity, sterility, weight gain and cell proliferation increasing the risk of cancer.[13] It is probable that the balancing effect of omega-3 on omega-6 may account for the therapeutic merits of fish-oil supplementation, although many studies link *essential* fats with serious health problems.

Conflicting studies are not unusual in a world where research is commissioned by those who can pay for it. Rarely done out of academic interest, research is expensive and the objective is ultimately to boost sales. Like most of us, science today has succumbed to the demands of the marketplace and is often used to promote economic interests. Journalists rarely read the original reports and are fed 'conclusions' by the industry, which inform the way research is reported in the media. A recent example is criticism of the Paleo diet in the mass media, based on a paper published by the National Academy of Sciences in America. Media reports misrepresented the findings, widely criticising the diet, to which the NAS has issued a rebuttal, but this is unlikely to attract much, if any, publicity. The truth is that today less than 12 per cent of medical journalism is accurate and 70 per cent of the information provided by drug companies for doctors is 'misleading'. This is why most people, who obtain their information from the mass media, believe low-fat diets to be healthy and saturated fat to be harmful.

In spite of what health experts may want us to think, extracted oils have only become available since WWII and PUFAs cause free-radical damage. If you thought Stone Age man wouldn't have wasted much time harvesting, grinding and fermenting grains, you might also be wondering if he would have bothered trying to extract oils from nuts, seeds and fish. What a time-consuming and frustrating task that would have been with only a pestle and mortar to hand. The advantage of the evolutionary model is that it can tell us much about traditional diets, and this is where we should look for information rather than media soundbites generated by the food and drug industries. Dr Weston Price found butter to be a staple in many traditional diets, so it is reasonable to assume that it would have been eaten by at least some of our Paleo ancestors too. Of the modern hunter-gatherers studied, those who didn't eat butter, ensured a good intake of fat-soluble vitamins from high-fat foods like fish, shellfish, eggs, organ meats, blubber from sea animals and insects.[14] Not one of the societies studied by Dr Weston Price consumed vegetable oils. From the Masai in Africa, who thrive on a diet of mostly milk, blood and beef, to the Inuit living off marine animals and blubber, there is no evidence of heart disease or indeed any degenerative disease. This is not surprising since saturated fats are essential for health. They:

- Strengthen cell membranes
- Incorporate calcium into bones
- Protect against heart disease
- Protect the liver from toxins
- Boost immunity and have anti-microbial properties
- Enhance omega-3 uptake.

However, the drive to promote cholesterol-lowering drugs like statins has ensured the cardio-protective effects of saturated fats are not widely known.

The importance of PUFAs has been the mainstay of medical and nutritional dogma for the last few decades and so it was with some trepidation that I decided to test this heresy out. I cut out polyunsaturated oils, stopped the fish oil supplements[*] and increased my saturated fat intake by eating coconut fat and raw, pastured butter. I have never looked back. Not for me the low-energy, middle-aged spread and liver spots that some of my colleagues are sporting.

In a paper published in January 2013, verbosely entitled 'Maternal plasma PUFA status in late pregnancy is associated with offspring body composition in childhood',[15] researchers were able accurately to predict fat mass of offspring based on maternal omega-6 status during pregnancy. In other words, mothers who were higher in omega-6 PUFAs gave birth to children who became fatter by the age of six. (The same correlation was not found to exist in respect of omega-3s.)

The idea that our diets should be high in carbohydrate and low in fat was first popularised in the 1960s and has influenced the way we eat ever since.[16] Based on conclusions drawn from the Sydney Heart Study carried out between 1966 and 1973, carbs suddenly became the cornerstone of a healthy diet. Modern methods of number crunching (computers) recently reanalysed the original data and, much to the surprise of the researchers, a

---

* Most fish oil supplements tend to contain only EPA (eicosapentaenoic acid – an omega-3 fat found in oily fish, egg yolks and meat) and DHA extracted from the whole fish using heat which can damage the fats. Green Pastures Cod Liver Oil uses a traditional fermentation process and only extracts oil from the liver. High in micronutrients and quinones, such as vitamins K and E and co-enzyme Q10, and containing all forms of natural vitamin A (rather than just beta carotene or retinol) this supplement is a whole food and replicates the cod liver oil eaten since Roman and Viking times but which dropped from favour after 1850 when heat made it possible to manufacture oil within minutes rather than hours.

completely different picture emerged. It is now evident that the conclusions drawn from the Sydney Heart Study were incorrect. Getting the maths wrong has spawned the high-carb/low-fat advice that has led many to their deaths from cardiovascular disease over the intervening years.

## Sat fat solution

Peat was the first to raise concerns about the safety of PUFAs and has long been a lone voice in his championing of saturated fats. It now seems that the tide is starting to turn as research is accumulating to vindicate his theories. Not that it's been welcomed by the pharmaceutical or food industries, as revoking previous guidelines can compromise professional credibility, not to mention the impact it would have on food buying and drug sales. In fact, since 2000 it has not been possible to publish any article criticising statins in a peer-reviewed journal.[18] Such an about-turn in policy would bring these industries crashing to a halt as the demand for low-fat foods dried up and the statin gravy train became derailed. For now, however, the industry in snake, sorry, nut, seed and fish oils continues to thrive as they are promoted as some universal panacea. Supplemented by almost everyone, from the pregnant to the menopausal and the hyperactive to the arthritic, extracted oils from nuts and seeds strike me as just another example of the industrialisation of food.

## Cholesterol – innocent bystander

Study after study has shown that a reduction in dietary cholesterol makes no difference to blood levels as the liver will simply make up any shortfall in the diet. Reducing consumption of white flour and sugar, however, does lower cholesterol levels, but before we get too excited it is important to realise that cholesterol levels naturally rise with age, and do not present health problems unless the cholesterol is rancid. As a saturated fat, we know that it is less likely to become rancid compared with PUFAs. In fact, as we shall shortly see, cholesterol has a protective effect against free radicals and may actually become elevated in response to a lack of nutrients in the diet and to environmental toxins.

Like saturated fat, cholesterol is essential for health. Needed to make bile and hormones, including insulin, and vitamin D, without it minerals cannot be used, calcium cannot get into bone, muscles lose tone, and immunity and fertility go down. As an antioxidant, cholesterol protects against brain damage, heart disease and cancer. In fact, the brain relies upon cholesterol to function and this is why statins are linked to dementia, depression and suicide. Serotonin, the feel-good chemical, prevents depression and insomnia but is useless without cholesterol. Memory and confusion can result from low levels of the memory chemical, acetylcholine, and this is why low cholesterol can cause dementia and Alzheimer's. Hopefully, as the detrimental impact of statins starts to become more widely known, the statin bandwagon will soon hit the buffers.

Rather than being the villain of the piece, cholesterol is used as a sort of Band-Aid to repair damaged blood vessels. Blood vessels become inflamed by our old friends, free radicals, and by viruses, and from autoantibody attack by the milk protein xanthine oxidase. A major cause of damage to arteries is from high blood sugar levels. Astoundingly, the advice given to cardiovascular patients today is to cut down on cholesterol, despite the fact that this would further raise the blood sugar, thus increasing inflammation. Nevertheless, this is standard medical practice – backed up by a high-carb diet, avoidance of red meat and a dose of statins.

Just what constitutes elevated cholesterol is unclear. The goal posts are moved regularly as the 'safe' reference range is reduced to dangerously low levels in a blatant bid to ensnare more into the statin net, regardless of the fact that 85 per cent of patients who suffer a heart attack have normal cholesterol levels. The cholesterol scam has been well documented in many books, including *Lipitor – Thief of Memory* and *Statin Drugs Side Effects*, both by Duane Graveline, former NASA doctor, astronaut and aerospace medical research scientist, whose brain was so befuddled on statins that he couldn't remember his own name or recognise his wife, symptoms that resolved when he stopped taking them.

As the unfortunate explorer and anthropologist Vilhjalmur Stefansson discovered, low-fat meat is toxic. As I described on page xxi, he and his colleague ran into problems for the first time in 11 years when they switched to low-fat meat. Dr McClelland, the scientist in charge of the study, wrote: 'At our request [Stefansson] began eating lean meat only, although he had previously noted, in the North, that very lean meat sometimes produced digestive disturbances. On the third day nausea and diarrhoea developed. When fat meat was added to the diet a full recovery was made in two days.'

This raises concerns regarding the modern interpretation of the Paleo diet which advocates eating lean meat and obtaining fat from nut and seed oils. Even if coconut oil, a saturated fat with many benefits to health, were included this would still present a problem since lack of organ meats would render such a diet nutritionally deficient in DHA and fat soluble vitamins. It is often forgotten that our Paleo ancestors lived an outdoor life and were exposed to more sunlight than we are, reducing the need for dietary sources of vitamin D.

### *Fat and weight*

Our bodies store excess energy as fat rather than protein, so it is obviously more logical to obtain our energy from fat as this is the body's preferred fuel source. This is one reason why it can be hard to lose weight by restricting calories without considering from which food groups the calories are derived. The body makes hormones out of fat. Hormones involved in blood sugar regulation, such as insulin, glucagon and cortisol, are essential for regulating weight and appetite. A good intake of fat has the additional advantage of reducing the temptation to over-eat as it provides a feeling of satiety, maintains stable blood sugar levels and reduces sweet cravings.

Studies at the Faculty of Medicine at the University of Geneva found that saturated and shorter chain fats discourage weight gain. Animal fats and coconut oil are slightly lower in calories than vegetable fats, coming in at 7.5 per gram as opposed to 9. Incidentally, fish oils are the most fattening, followed next by vegetable oils and olive oil respectively. So if you want to have more energy and reduce your risk of disease, try eating fatty meat, butter and coconut oil and get rid of any PUFAs lurking in your kitchen.

A weight problem is a symptom of a deranged metabolism, which includes insulin resistance, dysregulation of appetite hormones and compromised energy production in the cells. For these reasons, eating a high-fat diet can result in weight gain in the overweight. It is therefore necessary to optimise metabolic function so that the body is again able to burn fats for energy. Ways of doing this include exercise, intermittent fasting, low-carb diets and supplements to support cellular energy production.

## Agribusiness

The industrialisation of food has completely changed the nutrients in foods like meat and eggs. Cows eating a grain-based diet have omega-6 to -3 ratios exceeding 20:1 compared to grass-fed meat of around 3:1. Dr Cordain believes the ideal ratio to be closer to 1:2 or 1:1. The omega-3 content of grass-fed beef is 7 per cent of the total fat, compared with 1 per cent in grain-only fed beef.

Grass-fed beef is richer in vitamins and minerals and a fat

called 'CLA' or conjugated linoleic acid. Levels of CLA have been steadily diminishing in meat since grain feeding was introduced in the 1950s. Studies have shown this fat to be protective against cancer, obesity, diabetes and immunological disorders, and it is sometimes supplemented to dieters to promote weight loss. Today cows are routinely fed corn and soy oil because of their suppressive effect on thyroid hormones, with the specific intention of encouraging weight gain.[17] Unfortunately, the meat from these animals has the same effect on humans, and we now find ourselves in the ludicrous position of producing meat that contains vegetable oil.

### So what about eating Paleo today?

Assuming you do not intend including grubs and insects in your diet, and don't have access to wild meats, the Paleo diet would need to be adapted to satisfy your nutritional requirements from the foods available today. As we have seen, indigenous diets were high in saturated fat from organ meats and glands and some even included butter from grass-fed cows. Modern advocates of Paleo eating could run into trouble were they to rely solely on modern meat (which is bred to be leaner) to satisfy their need for fat soluble vitamins (A, D, E and K) and for DHA and CLA. Muscle meat is the least nutritious part of the animal. However, as a saturated animal fat, butter is a fat familiar to the body and rarely presents a problem if eaten raw.

The fat-soluble vitamins have to be eaten with fat or they cannot be utilised by the body. Native peoples studied by Dr Weston Price valued the butter of cows fed on rapidly growing green grass. The reason for this was due to its exceptionally high vitamin A content, though they were of course unaware of what the important factor was. Many studies have subsequently confirmed native wisdom in prizing foods rich in fat-soluble vitamins even though the existence of vitamins and the reasons they were beneficial were not understood. This phenomenon is well documented in Dr Weston A Price's *Nutrition and Physical Degeneration*. Vitamin A is known to come in at least 15 forms but the most well researched are **retinol**, which is found in animal fats, and **beta carotene**, which is found in plants, the most well-known example being carrots. Vegetarians claim that beta carotene is a good source of vitamin A, but it has recently been discovered that many people are poor converters of beta carotene to the active form, retinol, and furthermore this conversion is dependent on saturated fat. If your palms turn orange after drinking carrot juice, you are almost certainly unable to convert beta carotene to its active form. Minerals too have to be combined with fat-soluble vitamins before they can be assimilated, and Dr Weston Price believed that the fat-soluble vitamins were also necessary for the uptake of the water-soluble. As we have seen from Stefansson's experience (see page 6), meat is toxic unless combined with fat. Dr Weston Price believed the perfect bone structure, straight teeth and good complexions of the people he studied were due to their high intake of fat.

Researcher Roselind Wulzen identified what she termed 'anti-stiffness' factor in raw animal fat. Popularly known as the 'Wulzen factor', it protects from calcification of the joints, which causes progressive stiffness, a common problem in the elderly. Calves fed pasteurised milk seize up fairly quickly, developing joint stiffness and failing to thrive, symptoms which are quickly reversed with the addition of raw butterfat into their diets. Could it be that the arthritis which plagues the elderly today is simply the culmination of years of poor calcium metabolism resulting from a lifetime of drinking pasteurised milk?

Dr Weston Price also recognised something special in the organ meats and milk of grass-fed cows (and in some fish), which he called 'Activator X', which is now thought to be vitamin K2. Essential for mineral utilisation, it is nearly always found to be deficient in osteoporosis. Although it is one of the few nutrients not destroyed by pasteurisation, it is not found in cows that are not grass fed. It is possible that preventing intensively reared cows from grazing may have resulted in widespread vitamin K deficiency, driving the osteoporosis and arthritis epidemic in the elderly which is believed by the medical profession to be the inevitable result of having outlived the body's lifespan. This, however, does not stand up to scrutiny as modern-day hunter-gatherers tend to outlive their 'civilised' counterparts without the degenerative diseases that afflict us.

Calcium, a mineral almost everyone thinks they need to supplement thanks to milk-marketing hype, becomes bio-unavailable in the absence of co-factors, which include certain minerals and vitamins D and K. When this happens, the body will deposit it anywhere it can and this may include the joints (arthritis), the liver, the gall bladder or the kidneys (stones), or along the artery walls (atherosclerosis). Both these vitamins are often found to be low amongst the general population and, unless the individual is eating fatty, grass-fed meats, would also be likely to be deficient on a modern Paleo diet.

Arachidonic acid, a fat until recently dismissed as being pro-inflammatory and therefore best avoided, is now known to be important for the brain, cell membranes and the formation of anti-inflammatory (as well as pro-inflammatory) prostaglandins. Animal fats are the sole source of arachidonic acid.

### Fat and gall bladder disease

The gall bladder is a little pouch that sits below the liver and stores bile, essential for fat digestion. It is estimated that up to 95 per cent of us on the 'civilised' diet have stones in our livers, with the overspill being deposited in the gall bladder where it causes congestion and interferes with the release of bile. This results in an inability to digest fat. The majority of stones are calcium oxalate and form as a consequence of poor calcium metabolism – otherwise known as fat, vitamin and mineral deficiency. Following a low-fat diet is one of the most efficient methods of forming stones. The gall bladder is stimulated to release bile in response to the ingestion of dietary fat, and quickly becomes sludged-up when fat is in short supply. A high-carb diet, especially if it contains high-fructose corn syrup, will also do the trick as fructose and unused sugars are converted to fat in the liver, where they cause congestion.

Despite the fact that only 1 to 4 per cent of patients have symptoms, gall bladder removal is the new kid on the block when it comes to unnecessary, high-tech surgery. Since the development of keyhole surgery, affectionately referred to by doctors as 'lap choly' (short for laporoscopic cholecystectomy), gall bladders can now be whipped out via an incision an inch long. Since this procedure was introduced in 1989, cholecystectomies have increased, with 750,000 Americans each year being duped into believing they would be better off without a gall bladder. To my knowledge, medical advice following surgery does not include supplementation with fat-soluble vitamins, bile- and fat-digesting enzymes and the consumption of saturated fat. In fact, most patients are told to eat a low-fat diet and since carbs can be converted to fat and stored in the liver this advice would seem unhelpful to say the least. Although the liver can drip feed bile into the gut in the absence of a gall bladder, surgery almost always increases liver congestion and results in deficiencies of fat and the fat-soluble vitamins. The reduction in fat available to the brain and nervous system following cholecystectomy would be likely to increase the risk of multiple health problems including cognitive impairment. This has been well documented in the book *Lipitor – Thief of Memory* by Duane Graveline, a former NASA doctor who was unable to recognise his own wife when taking statins. Cholesterol is also needed to make the myelin sheath that covers the nerves. In addition, since bile is vital for the health of the intestine the risk of colon cancer increases by 50 per cent unless steps such as those outlined above are implemented. The gall bladder seems to have been another victim of the modern health police, as a low intake of dietary fat fails to stimulate the release of bile, which can stagnate, causing infection or inflammation and this is a common reason for its removal. Supplements and herbs exist that will dissolve stones and there are natural methods, such as liver flushes, for cleansing the liver and gall bladder which would seem a less radical alternative to surgery.

### The Urban Caveman diet and fat

My concern about the fat intake of the modern Paleo diet was one of the reasons why I developed my own variant – the Urban Caveman diet. Since fat appears to be the rate-limiting factor when it comes to health, I think it is important to include raw butters, which are generally well tolerated even by those with allergies to dairy. (Raw, or unpasteurised, butters can be ordered online or you can find producers local to you by visiting www.naturalfoodfinder. co.uk and www.bigbarn.co.uk.) Since protein is toxic without fat, and because modern meats are leaner, I think properly produced butter represents a beneficial addition to the diet. Assuming that anyone considering a Paleo-style diet is motivated by a desire to improve health, this should override any qualms about whether the foods were part of the ancestral diet.

## Quick recap

- A saturated fat is stable when heated whereas a polyunsaturated fat is liable to become rancid.
- Polyunsaturated fats could promote disease as they weaken the cell membranes and could also encourage weight gain due to their inhibiting effect on energy.
- It is healthy to eat more saturated fat.
- Protein needs fat for its metabolism.

## Personal health check

Could you be **low in fat**? Tick any of the following that apply to you:

| | | | |
|---|---|---|---|
| | Sweet craving | | Low energy |
| | Dry skin | | Hair loss |
| | Stiff joints | | Low-fat diet now or in past |
| | Gall bladder problems or gall bladder removed | | Light or clay-coloured stools |
| | Nausea when eating fat | | Tension headache at base of skull |
| | Sunburn easily | | Muscles easily tired |
| | Dandruff | | Itchy, flaky skin on feet |
| | Osteoporosis | | Osteoarthritis |

In addition to the fat fiasco, one of the other perils of the Western diet is the rise in sugar consumption. First introduced four centuries ago, sugar is now consumed in gargantuan amounts by most people today. What that means for your health is set out in graphic detail in the next chapter.

# Chapter 8

# Sugar beat

Sugar is an anti-nutrient. Pure, white and deadly, to quote Professor John Yudkin, were it to be introduced today it would not be licensed as a food. It contains no fibre, no minerals, no proteins, no fats and no enzymes. Every time you eat sugar your body has to leech calcium, sodium, potassium, zinc, chromium and magnesium from your bones in order to metabolise it, and to buffer your blood against its acidity. This is why the regular consumption of sugar is known to cause osteoporosis. America and the UK are the world's two largest consumers of sugar.

In spite of the fact that most people are actively trying to reduce their intake, sugar consumption continues to rise. Routinely added to cold meats, sausages, bacon and nearly all processed foods, including savoury dishes like pizza, most of the sugar you eat today will be hidden.

Research published in 2007[1] showed refined sugar to be more addictive than cocaine. Its chemical formula is $C12H22O11$ (12 carbon, 22 hydrogen and 11 oxygen atoms). Cocaine is $C17H21NO4$ (17 carbon, 21 hydrogen, 1 nitrogen and 4 oxygen atoms). From a practical point of view there is very little difference between the two. A study on cocaine-addicted rats found that they preferentially chose sugar water over cocaine and that they were more willing to work for sugar than cocaine! The researchers deduced that excessive stimulation from sugar triggers the reward centre in the hypothalamus, overriding willpower and resulting in addiction, compulsive eating and obesity.

First cultivated 8,000 years ago[2] in the Pacific, sugar was transported to other parts of the globe where traders quickly learned to extract it from the cane. The first record of sugar addiction was recorded in 1573 by a German botanist who observed the Turks and Moors to be in the habit of cutting '…one piece of saccharum after another and chew and eat them openly everywhere in the street without shame! …in this way they accustom themselves to gluttony and are no longer the intrepid fighters they had formerly been.' At that time, due to its addictive nature,[3] sugar was as valuable as gemstones, but the market for sugar quickly became insatiable, and so slavery was introduced to meet the demand.

Sugar was first brought to Europe around 1700, when the average intake per capita went from zero to four pounds per year. By the 1950s, average annual consumption in the UK was 38 pounds and has risen by 31 per cent over the last two decades to 65 pounds per person, per year,[4] or 1.25 pounds per week. As the public wises up to the need to reduce their sugar intake, the industry has been forced to create new outlets, hence the trend away from 'visible' to 'invisible' sugar.

Its presence is not always apparent as many names are used to disguise it. Generally, any ingredient ending in 'ose' is likely to be a sugar – for example, dextrose, lactose, sucrose, fructose and glucose. The list below gives the most commonly found sugars. However, as far as the body is concerned, there is no distinction between different types of sugar, so honey or molasses would be processed in the same way as white sugar, and in fact any carbohydrate will eventually end up as sugar. How long it takes is determined by its 'glycaemic load' (see page 80).

The following are names used for the sugars added to processed foods. Look out for them, know what they are and avoid them if you can:

Amasake

Apple sugar

Barbados sugar

Bark sugar

Barley malt

Barley malt syrup

Beet sugar

Brown rice syrup

Brown sugar

Cane juice

Cane sugar

Caramelised foods

Carbitol

Carmel coloring

Carmel sugars

Concentrated fruit juice

Corn sweetener

Corn syrup

Date sugar

Dextrin

Dextrose

Diglycerides

Disaccharides

D-tagalose

Evaporated cane juice

Florida crystals

Fructooligosaccharides (FOS)

Fructose

Fruit juice concentrate

Galactose.

Glucitol

Glucoamine

Gluconolactone

Glucose

Glucose polymers

Glucose syrup

Glycerides

Glycerine

Glycerol

Glycol

Hexitol

High-fructose corn syrup

Honey

Inversol

Invert sugar

Isomalt

Karo syrups

Lactose

Levulose

'Light' sugar

'Lite' sugar

Malitol

Malt dextrin

Malted barley

Maltodextrins

Maltodextrose

Maltose

Malts

Mannitol

Mannose

Maple syrup

Microcrystalline cellulose

Molasses

Monoglycerides

Monosaccarides

Nectars

Neotame

Pentose

Polydextrose

Polyglycerides

Powdered sugar

Raisin juice

Raisin syrup

Raw sugar

Ribose rice syrup

Rice malt

Rice sugar

Rice sweeteners

Rice syrup solids

Saccharides

Sorbitol

Sorghum

Sucanat

Sucanet

Sucrose

Sugar cane

Trisaccharides

Turbinado sugar

Unrefined sugar

White sugar

Xylitol

Zylose

In 1979, Professor Philip James, deputy director of the Medical Research Council Clinical Nutrition Department at Cambridge University, recommended a reduction in sugar consumption. However, James's findings were criticised by none other than the British Nutrition Foundation – which is not all that surprising, considering it is funded by the food industry. 'The sugar industry has learned the tricks of the tobacco industry,' said James. 'Confuse the public. Produce experts who disagree, try to dilute the message, indicate that there are extremists like me involved in public health.'[5]

Other examples abound, as you are no doubt starting to realise, such as the prestigiously named International Life Sciences Institute, which sounds like a reputable academic institution, until you discover that it is primarily owned by Coca Cola, whose soft drink contains 39 grams of sugar per can or 9.75 teaspoons.[6] Incidentally, Sprite comes in at 38 grams and Pepsi at 41 grams, and the sugar effects are further exacerbated by the addition of caffeine, which is often added to many soft drinks. Sports drinks fare no better, as they frequently contain the same levels of sugar as other soft drinks.

The blood stream of an adult should contain between one and two teaspoons of glucose *in total*, which equates to roughly one part per thousand.[7] A chocolate bar is likely to contain more than 16 teaspoons of sugar, which represents quite a whack when fed to a small child. The average sugar consumption in the US is around 70 teaspoons per day, and the UK is quickly catching up. The body works hard to maintain what is called 'homeostatic balance' – not only of sugar, but also fluid, acid / alkaline levels, mineral salts and so on. This means that the sugar level shouldn't deviate more than a fraction from the ideal concentration, and this is why any dip or rise in sugar levels provokes symptoms. If the blood sugar becomes too low, the adrenals respond by producing stress hormones that pull glucose out of the cells and into the blood stream. *This is a major cause of panic attacks.*

Conversely, if the blood sugar becomes too high, the pancreas and liver produce insulin and glucose tolerance factor (GTF) respectively to clear the sugar from the blood, which it does by dumping it into the cells where it is stored, usually in the form of fat. Even a slight fluctuation in sugar levels puts the body into a crisis state requiring an immediate response as sugar can be lethal at high levels, and both high and low blood sugar can eventually result in loss of consciousness. It is impossible to overstate the effect of sugar on mood and behaviour. The brain is particularly vulnerable as the body is designed to ensure the brain is functional even if blood sugar levels are low throughout the rest of the body. This means that the brain will be flooded with sugar if levels become too high, which can result in mental confusion, mood instability and even criminal behaviour. When too low, only the aggressive part of the brain remains functional, and drops in blood sugar are responsible for some of the road rage and aggressive behaviours we see today. The effects of fluctuating blood sugar on the brain are explored in the book *Diet, Crime and Delinquency* by Dr Alexander Schauss.

## The big breakfast binge

If like millions of others you start the day with a carbohydrate fix like cereal or toast, accompanied by margarine and marmalade, washed down with a coffee made with skimmed (high sugar) milk your breakfast would be almost exclusively comprised of sugar and devoid of good fats. Often combined with caffeine to kick-start the adrenals, a cereal-based breakfast ensures that the blood sugar level reaches dangerous levels before you have even left the house. In fact, this artificial, adrenalinised 'energy' is often the only energy many people have. Regular sugar top-ups are required throughout the day, so this is a high-maintenance diet. Over time it will exhaust the pancreas, liver and adrenals, which have to be on red-alert so they can swing into action with every fluctuation in blood sugar. In this scenario, blood glucose tends to lurch from being disproportionately high to hypoglycaemic as the over-reacting endocrine glands attempt to impose some degree of homeostatic balance. The drops in blood glucose are experienced as the characteristic mid-morning slump when another sugar fix is needed, such as a coffee or carbohydrate-based pick-me-up, or a crafty cigarette, whilst the highs can make you hyperactive but unproductive.

Unstable blood sugar causes peaks and troughs in energy, resulting in bursts of hyperactivity alternating with drowsiness, irritability alternating with brain fog, and can even provoke mood disorders. Night time isn't usually much fun either, as high levels of stress hormones attempting to maintain adequate blood sugar levels whilst you sleep may initially make it hard to drop off, or cause wakefulness in the small hours. At three o'clock in the morning, a hypoglycaemic brain awash with stress hormones will make you feel anxious about everything, drawing you into a vicious cycle of escalating anxiety and insomnia.

Getting up in the morning usually presents a challenge as well, as you may not be able to function until you have cranked-up your blood sugar – hence the breakfast, and thus the whole cycle starts all over again. Eating a high-carb breakfast sets the stage for sweet cravings throughout the day, beating the resolve of the most resolute dieter, whilst a fat and protein breakfast would have a stabilising effect on blood sugar and energy levels. Incidentally, an aversion to breakfast or early morning nausea can also be a sign of low blood sugar.

The blood sugar see-saw places a great strain on the body, robbing it of nutrients whilst the cells are alternately flooded with or starved of glucose. Pumping out large quantities of insulin puts a great strain on the pancreas. As most of its work involves the production of digestive juices and enzymes, less than 1 per cent of pancreatic cells are designed to produce insulin. 'Healthy' cereal bars tend to be as high in sugar as chocolate, and breakfast cereals are really a form of confectionary. Table 3 shows the nutritional content of some popular cereals.

You will see that none of the cereals provide any appreciable amount of fat, apart from the damaging trans fats, which were found in Corn Pops and Honey Smacks. The highest sugar content was dished up by Kellogg's Raisin Bran Crunch with Smart Start Healthy Heart scoring second place in the sugar stakes with a whopping 17 grams, or over four teaspoons per serving! This *unhealthy* start to the day was also the highest in calories, weighing in with 230, and the highest in carbohydrate. More worryingly, it also contains HFCS (high fructose corn syrup), about which more below. Since there is ample research linking sugar to cardio-vascular disease and HFCS to high blood pressure and elevations in blood fats, it would be interesting to know by what criteria anyone could possibly consider such a cereal to be cardio-protective. Unfortunately, the health conscious consumer might be fooled into purchasing these cereals, having been deceived by clever branding into presuming that bran is good because of its fibre content, and that raisins have replaced the sugar. However, raisins, in common with other dried fruits, are, in fact, a potent source of concentrated sugar and for this reason are not recommended on the Paleo diet.

An article in the *Daily Mail* in April 2010 entitled 'Named and Shamed: The cereals with more sugar than a bowl of ice cream', reported a survey in the consumer magazine *Which* that found some cereals contained more salt than ready-salted crisps, and concluded that, '…the vast majority of breakfast cereals [are] of "poor nutrition".' Using guidelines from the Food Standards Agency, a whopping 92 per cent contained higher than the recommended levels of sugar considered acceptable. With the majority of kids and drivers tanked up on this early morning sugar binge, I'm glad I am not on the roads in the rush hour.

A food can never be neutral in terms of its effect on our health – it is either good for us or it is bad. The *Mail* compared the sugar

| Cereal | Serving size: 1 cup | Calories | Total fat (grams) | Saturated fat (grams) | |
|---|---|---|---|---|---|
| Kellogg's Cornflakes | 1 | 100 | 0 | 0 | |
| Kellogg's Rice Crispies | 1.25 | 120 | 0 | 0 | |
| Kellogg's Frosted Flakes | 0.75 | 110 | 0 | 0 | |
| Kellogg's Frosted Krispies | 0.75 | 110 | 0 | 0 | |
| Kellogg's Special K (Red Berries) | 1 | 110 | 0 | 0 | |
| Kellogg's Honey Smacks | 0.75 | 100 | 0.5 | 0 | |
| General Mills Wheaties | 0.75 | 100 | 0.5 | 0 | |
| Kellogg's Special K | 1 | 120 | 0.5 | 0 | |
| Kellogg's All-Bran | 0.5 | 80 | 1 | 0 | |
| Post Shredded Wheat | 47 | 200 | 1 | 0 | |
| Genreal Mills Multi Grain Cheerios | 1 | 110 | 1 | 0 | |
| Kellogg's Raisin Bran Crunch | 1 | 190 | 1 | 0 | |
| General Mills Cocoa Puffs | 0.75 | 110 | 1.5 | 0 | |
| Quaker Life | 0.75 | 120 | 1.5 | 0 | |
| General Mills Honey Nut Cheerios | 0.75 | 110 | 1.5 | 0 | |
| General Mills Cheerios | 1 | 100 | 2 | 0 | |
| Kellogg's Smart Start Healthy Heart | 1.25 | 230 | 3 | 0.5 | |
| General Mills Oatmeal Crisp Crunch Almond | 1 | 220 | 5 | 0.5 | |

**Table 3:** Nutritional content of breakfast cereals
Ref: www.acaloriecounter.com/breakfastcereal
(reproduced with permission)

| Carbs (grams) | Fibre (grams) | Sugar (grams) | Protein (grams) | Trans fats | HFCS (high fructose corn syrup) |
|---|---|---|---|---|---|
| 24 | 1 | 2 | 2 | No | Yes |
| 29 | 0 | 3 | 2 | No | Yes |
| 27 | 1 | 11 | 1 | No | Yes |
| 27 | 0 | 12 | 1 | No | Yes |
| 25 | 1 | 10 | 3 | No | Yes |
| 24 | 1 | 15 | 2 | Yes | No |
| 22 | 3 | 4 | 3 | No | No |
| 22 | 1 | 4 | 7 | No | Yes |
| 23 | 10 | 6 | 4 | No | Yes |
| 37 | 6 | 0 | 5 | No | No |
| 23 | 3 | 6 | 2 | No | No |
| 45 | 4 | 20 | 3 | No | Yes |
| 23 | 1 | 12 | 1 | No | No |
| 25 | 2 | 6 | 3 | No | NO |
| 22 | 2 | 9 | 3 | No | No |
| 20 | 3 | 1 | 3 | No | No |
| 46 | 5 | 17 | 7 | No | Yes |
| 46 | 4 | 16 | 6 | No | Yes |

content of cereals with one serving of Tesco's Dark Chocolate Fudge Brownie Ice Cream, which contained 11.6 grams (nearly four teaspoons) of sugar. This turned out to be substantially less than was found in Raisin Bran Crunch and Smart Start Healthy Heart. Cereals tested, which included Kellogg's Frosties, and Crunchy Nut, Morrisons Coco Pops Moons, Kellogg's Ricicles and Nestle Cookie Crisp amongst others, found that one 40 gram bowl, excluding milk, would provide on average 14.5 grams of sugar, converting into about three-and-a-half teaspoons. This would be enough to push the body into a crisis state because it has to act quickly to get the sugar out of circulation to prevent tissue damage. It generally achieves this by converting it to fat and storing it. Although this is likely to make you overweight, it is a short-term solution to protect against other health problems, including cancer, which thrives on sugar.

Studies have shown that even fruit juice can raise the blood sugar to dangerously high levels. Sugar kills up to 25 per cent of immune cells, and it can take 24 hours to replace them. This means that if you are eating sugar every day, your immune system may be functioning at three-quarters below capacity.

According to an article in the *British Medical Journal*, 'Sugar is *as dangerous as tobacco* (and) should be classified as a hard drug, for it is harmful and addictive.'[8] 'As dangerous as tobacco'? It is handed out willy-nilly by nursery schools, parents and teachers in reward for good work or as bribery to behave, or just because it's break time. Like the alcoholic who is habituated to regular fixes, children are being conditioned to need regular doses of sugar, and as a result are becoming fatter, lower in energy and at risk of degenerative disease.

At children's parties the sugar orgy reaches Bacchanalian proportions. The modern children's party revs kids up to a state of hyperactivity and manic over-excitement, which often continues into the night as they bounce off the bedroom walls instead of sleeping. So commonplace is the problem of sugar poisoning amongst the young, that parents who actively try to limit the sugar intake of their offspring are frequently confronted by obstacles at every turn. From undermining and colluding grandparents who sneak sweets to their 'deprived' grandchildren, to the bemused teacher who has been left without stick or carrot, or the unappreciative child who resents being singled out and denied the pleasures afforded to his peers, it is a brave parent who tries, Canute-style, to stand against the sugar tide engulfing this generation of children.

Our tastes and future health are determined at a very young age. Sugar addiction not only increases the risk of addictions generally but sows the seeds of poor health and obesity. Parents and teachers would not dream of offering cigarettes or alcohol to the children in their care but think nothing of giving them sweets, which are just as damaging. The lack of awareness is truly staggering, especially in a society that claims to be health conscious.

Not only are the young assaulted by confectionery, but modern fruits have been bred to taste sweeter, with supermarkets preferentially stocking the sweeter varieties. Often irradiated and laced with pesticides, diced sweet fruits like grapes and melons are often displayed near the supermarket check-out masquerading as a healthy way to placate a child in a queue. Labelled as a part of your 'five-a-day' – another arbitrary figure dreamt up by marketing rather than science – parents are enticed into buying another sugar fix.

## Baby bloomers

Research suggests that our need for sweetness is greatest during growth, but prior to the industrialisation of food, children were naturally exposed to a variety of different tastes which included bitter, savoury and sour. However, weaning on to manufactured baby foods encourages only the development of a taste for sweetness, as baby foods contain added sucrose (sugar) and are frequently made from concentrated fruits and caramelised vegetables. Such is the encroachment of the food industry into our lives that it may not have occurred to the modern parent that s/he could purée a fresh fruit herself or mash a vegetable, having been encouraged to believe that baby food comes out of jars. However, a 21 millilitre jar of fruit baby food will contain an average of 33 grams of sugar, which is the equivalent of just over eight teaspoons. Savoury purées are also very sweet. For example, there are three teaspoons of sugar in a 213 millilitre jar of sweet potato, and an average of one teaspoon in a meat dish.

Processed baby foods are the products of an industrialised process similar to pasteurisation, which involves reheating the already cooked food under jar pressure to around 121 degrees centigrade, or higher, for 40 minutes, ensuring the destruction of any vitamins it might originally have contained. Heating to 121 degrees centigrade also alters the structure of the proteins, which then may not be recognised by the immune system, thus increasing the risk of allergies. Intensive heat treatment is used to sterilise the food and is necessary for mass production; but who wants to feed their baby sterilised food? Exposure to such intense heat additionally alters the consistency,[9] taste and colour of the food, and *caramelises the sugars in the fruit and vegetables,* turning them to sugar. In 2006 there was a move to legally reduce the amount of sugar in baby foods from the existing maximum of 30 per cent to 10. However, this was blocked by the US and the EU. Many health-conscious parents may be inclined to feed their children yoghurts instead of desserts, assuming they are less sweet, but which in reality may be sweeter as many are one-fifth sugar. Frozen yoghurts are usually just desserts to which some beneficial bacteria have been added.

Follow-on formula milks are also incredibly sweet[10] and may contain up to 60 per cent more sugar than ordinary milk, which may explain the correlation between bottle-feeding and obesity. Ruth Randall,[11] policy director of the Baby Milk Action Group, says that a bottle-fed baby consumes 30,000[12] more calories within the first eight months of its life, compared with his breast-fed counterpart.

## Hidden sugars

'Lite' dairy produce may be virtually fat-free, but the fat will have been replaced by sugars, including artificial sweeteners and fructose, which is even sweeter than sucrose. Even foods that may appear at first glance to be savoury can also be laced with sugar, but this may not be obvious from the label. Crisps are often sweetened with aspartame, and more upmarket crisps may look as if they only have 'sea salt and black pepper flavouring',[13] but often contain the milk sugar lactose. The word 'flavouring' means nothing, as any additive could be described as 'flavouring' but is likely to include MSG or monosodium glutamate, a protein that can cause hyperactivity and which requires good levels of vitamin B6 to process. Processed cheeses, especially those marketed for children, usually contain sugar from skimmed milk powders.

Neil Rigby, director of policy at the International Obesity Taskforce,[14] has been quoted as saying: 'We are raising our children in the sweet shop...the food industry has some 30,000 varieties of chemical powder to tweak their artificial ingredients in other products to make them sweet. Why do they add sugars to savoury products? Presumably because their research tells them children like it, and it sells.' And sells it does, from the confectionery industry to the pharmaceutical syrups that are used to treat the ensuing diseases.

And we are eating more and more of it. Analysis from till receipts of public spending trends revealed the following changes over a one-year period between 2005 and 2006[15] in the UK:

- Soft drinks up by 34 per cent
- Cakes up by 2 per cent

- Chilled juices and fruit juices up 30 per cent
- Chocolate biscuits down by 9 per cent
- Chocolate confectionery up 5 per cent from £1.6 billion in 2005 to £1.7 billion in 2005.

Today the figures are truly staggering. By the age of seven, children in Britain are eating an average of half a kilo of sugary foods daily.[16] By the age of 15, boys are feeding a habit of nearly 80 pounds per year, the equivalent of 1,000 cans of cola or 11,800 cubes of sugar. It is thought that the figures could actually be much higher, since they were based on food diaries, and it is known that there is a tendency to under-estimate by about 34 per cent. However, encouraging the industry to reduce the amount of sugar in processed foods is not going to be easy. Sugar adds bulk,[17] prolongs shelf-life and is addictive. So today, the food industry has come up with 'sweetness modifiers', a new class of additive that may simply appear on the label as 'flavouring'. 'Sweetness modifiers' are chemicals that prevent taste receptors on the tongue from registering sweetness, and are recommended for savoury foods such as meats, cheese and salad dressings. The ingenuity of the food industry knows no bounds.

Our indigenous diet would have contained no sugar at all, apart from the natural sweetness of some fruits. Sugar kills off beneficial gut bacteria and encourages the growth of unwanted microbes like yeasts. Before 1700, we did not eat it. Furthermore, our fruits were lower in natural sugars, and honey would have been a very occasional treat, dependent upon someone having been brave enough to have extracted it from a beehive. Since sugar is anti-nutrient, nutritional deficiencies *always* accompany its consumption.

## Sugar and the liver

One of the problems with eating sugar is that it requires no digestion, so can flood the blood stream directly from the stomach and small intestine. However, this is a fast-food delivery system which bypasses all the protective mechanisms for keeping the blood sugar level stable. The liver is designed to make glucose out of fat or protein by a process called 'gluconeogenesis'. The advantage of this system is that the liver modifies glucose output according to demand, so it can gradually be released into the blood stream in accordance with our needs. This prevents the highs and lows associated with sugar consumption and this is why eliminating sugar can stabilise mood and energy. However, when first weaning off sugar, the initial response is likely to be one of fatigue because it can take a week of so for the body to get used to the idea that there is no longer a steady supply of sugar coming in. Until the liver has racked up its own sugar production, low energy, cravings and brain fog may result. However, increasing your intake of saturated fat like butter and coconut oil, and intermittent fasting, can help improve sensitivity to insulin and maintain blood glucose levels.

A common trap many people fall into is of simply replacing sugar with something else that will raise the blood sugar level, such as cigarettes, alcohol, tea, coffee, 'diet' drinks or fruit. Remember, you are dealing with addiction here. I have seen clients who believed they had given up sugar but were guzzling sweet fruits or drinking liquid sugar in the form of fruit juices.

## Sugar and obesity

The hypothalamus is a gland in the brain that monitors blood sugar and hormonal levels so that it can respond to an increase or decrease in demand according to activity levels. Continued saturation with excessively high levels of sugar could 'burn out' the glucose or insulin receptors on its cell membranes. Starved of glucose, it would be likely to conclude that the blood sugar was too low, and switch on the hunger hormones. Irresistible sugar cravings and insatiable appetite would lock the hapless victim in a binge/diet cycle and escalating weight gain. Anyone on this treadmill wouldn't go long enough without a sugar fix to experience a drop in blood sugar, so would be blissfully unaware of the hormonal and nutritional chaos daily ravaging his body, simply assuming it is due to 'a sweet tooth' and attributing his lowered energy and weight gain to ageing or lack of exercise.

## Insulin resistance

Insulin is a hormone produced in the pancreas in response to a rise in blood glucose. It helps maintain stable blood sugar levels by transporting the glucose into cells. However, a high-carbohydrate diet will stimulate an increased output of insulin, and when this happens the cells can eventually become unresponsive to it. This is known as **insulin resistance**. And if fat cells become insulin resistant, it becomes almost impossible to lose weight.

**Table 4:** Sugar content of common foods (in teaspoons)

| Food | Teaspoons | Food | Teaspoons |
|------|-----------|------|-----------|
| One sweet | 1 | One slice of cake | 4 |
| One sweet biscuit | 1 | One portion of jelly | 4 |
| One can soft drink | 12 | One glass of cordial | 5 |
| One glass of fruit juice | 3 | Two squares of chocolate | 1 |
| One teaspoon of jam | ½ | One scoop of ice-cream | 1.5 |
| One ice lolly | 5 | | |

Insulin resistance is common today and underlies many health problems. Known as the 'fat-storage hormone', its output needs to kept within narrow limits. Below is a list of some diseases directly linked to insulin resistance. It reads like a roll call of 21st-century health problems:

- **Acne**: Blackheads are one of the first sign that insulin levels are too high.
- **Addictions**: All addictions are a form of self-medicating and stimulants can raise the blood sugar.
- **Alzheimer's disease**: Now sometimes referred to as 'type 3 diabetes' as insulin resistance in the brain is a key feature.
- **Arthritis**: Bio-unavailable calcium raises insulin levels and sugar causes inflammation.
- **Asthma**: Toxic blood from a congested liver irritates the lungs, and sugar causes inflammation.
- **Cardiovascular disease**: There is always insulin resistance causing inflammation in the blood vessels, upsetting mineral levels for healthy heart function and causing fats to be stored in the liver and blood vessels.
- **Cancer**: Cancer cells thrive on sugar.
- **Dysbiosis**: This is an imbalance in gut ecology. Sugar feeds the pathogenic microbes and kills beneficial bacteria.
- **Eczema**: As asthma.
- **Headaches**: These are often triggered by low blood sugar and also linked to liver congestion, which can be the result of fat deposition stimulated by insulin.
- **High cholesterol**: Insulin resistance causes cholesterol levels to rise as insulin stimulates the conversion of unused sugar to fat.
- **Hyperactivity**: The brain becomes overstimulated when flooded with sugar and aggressive when sugar levels drop.
- **Infections**: Sugar destroys 50 per cent of immune cells and it takes our bodies five hours to replace them. It also destroys vitamin C.
- **Learning difficulties and behavioural problems**:

Fluctuations in blood sugar alternately over-stimulate and then depress brain function.

- **Migraine**: This can be brought on by a drop in blood sugar. There is nearly always liver congestion.

- **Menopausal symptoms**: Unstable blood sugar can cause many menopausal symptoms including hot flushes.

- **Mood disorders/Bipolar/Depression**: Fluctuations in blood sugar alternately saturate and then depress glucose levels in the brain making it difficult to maintain balanced levels of brain chemicals (neurotransmitters).

- **Myopia (short-sightedness)**: This may be a symptom of insulin resistance.

- **Non-alcoholic fatty liver disease (NAFLD)**: This may be initiated by high-fructose corn syrup; unused sugar is converted to fat under the stimulation of insulin.

- **Obesity, weight problems and eating disorders**: Insulin resistance upsets hypothalamic function which is where the pleasure centre is located. Any addiction is an attempt to artificially stimulate the pleasure centre. Obesity results from insulin resistance as the body is unable to burn fat for energy whilst insulin causes sugar to be stored as fat.

- **Osteopenia and osteoporosis**: Sugar is very acidic and causes calcium to be pulled out of bones to alkalise the blood. Insulin levels rise in the presence of bio-unavailable calcium.

- **Panic attacks, anxiety, insomnia**: When the blood sugar level drops the adrenal glands pump out stress hormones like adrenaline and cortisone, producing the feeling of fear.

- **PMT**: Premenstrual tension is often the result of insulin resistance worsened by elevations in oestrogen and magnesium deficiency. A craving for sweets pre-menstrually is often a symptom of magnesium deficiency. Zinc is needed to balance hormones but may be diverted into making insulin instead.

- **Polycystic ovarian syndrome (PCOS)/Hormonal imbalance/ Hirsuitism in women**: If insulin is not able to dock on to cells, it stimulates the release of eggs in the ovaries. It also lowers levels of a hormone produced in the liver that breaks down testosterone. In girls this can cause excess body hair, which often accompanies PCOS.
- **Urinary tract infections or cystitis**: Sugar can irritate the bladder wall and cause overgrowth of pathogenic bacteria.
- **Yeast overgrowth**: Yeasts in the gut can mop up sugars, protecting the blood stream from being flooded with sugar. A high sugar diet will inevitably cause yeast overgrowth.

## Frankinsyrup and the liver

Unused sugar, particularly fructose, is converted to fat and deposited in the liver where it can lead to NAFLD, or 'non-alcoholic fatty liver disease', as noted in the list. Until recently, NAFLD was only observed in alcoholics, but it is now affecting children under 10 years old. The liver carries out over 500 functions which it cannot do efficiently if it is clogged up with fatty deposits. This can result in gall bladder disease and difficulty breaking down bilirubin from old red blood cells, causing yellowing of the skin. When the liver becomes engorged there may be a backwash into the lymph system, causing the development of cellulite; alternatively, toxic bile may enter the stomach during the night causing bad breath, morning nausea or heartburn. In fact, almost every system of the body could be affected as good liver function is fundamental to hormonal balance, detoxification, blood sugar regulation, excretion of toxins, the conversion of fats to energy, and so on. Moreover, if there is a log-jam in the liver, the kidneys may have to step in and start cleaning up the blood, causing headaches, including migraines, urinary tract infections (cystitis), skin problems, asthma, neck and shoulder stiffness, low energy and brain fog.

One of the reasons for the epidemic of NAFLD is thought to have been the introduction of high-fructose corn syrup (HFCS) in the '70s, welcomed by the food industry as an even cheaper preservative than sugar. It has subsequently been realised that as far as the liver is concerned, there is no difference between HFCS and fructose, the naturally occurring sugar in fruit, as they are both broken down by the same pathway, producing a toxic intermediary called aldehyde. HFCS can set the body up for obesity as it disrupts appetite and metabolism and plunges the body into fat storage mode.

Carbohydrate is made up of carbon, hydrogen and oxygen – this is the reason for its name. The blood sugar level will spike after eating grains and legumes, but this does not happen after eating vegetables, although they are high in carbs. So, if you are looking for ways of boosting energy and reducing your weight it would make sense to eliminate grains and legumes from your diet, unless properly prepared by soaking, fermenting or sprouting. Sprouting is something anyone can easily do at home. Simply soak the beans overnight in water and then place in a sprouter and water twice daily. There are many books dedicated to sprouting and fermenting as these are methods favoured by raw foodists. Such methods of preparation reduce levels of phytic acid and enzyme inhibitors whilst increasing the nutritional content of the bean.

## Quick recap

- Sugar is linked to osteoporosis as its acidity causes minerals to be leached out of the bones.
- Insulin is the hormone needed to get sugar into cells.
- The pancreas's main job is to produce digestive enzymes and juices.

- Sugar is linked to anxiety and anger as a rise in blood sugar can overstimulate the brain and dips in blood sugar can cause irritability, anxiety and aggression.

## Personal health check

Could you have **unstable blood sugar**? Tick any box that applies to you.

| | | | |
|---|---|---|---|
| | Low energy on waking | | Dips in energy during the day |
| | Craving for sweet foods | | Frequent need to pass urine |
| | Thirst | | Difficulty sleeping |
| | Anxiety | | Jittery or irritable if meal skipped |
| | Panic attacks | | Sleepy in the afternoon |
| | Excessive appetite | | Crave pick-me-ups |
| | Awaken a few hours after falling asleep | | Fatigue relieved by eating |
| | Headache if meal skipped | | Family members with diabetes |
| | Overweight | | |

# Chapter 9

# Vegetarianism – dicing with diet

Three decades ago vegetarianism was virtually obligatory for anyone interested in health, whilst others gave up meat for moral and ecological reasons. I myself was one of them. I didn't eat meat or fish for 20 years, eight of which were vegan. Prompted by a love of animals and horror at the way they were treated, I considered myself well informed, and believed I was benefiting not only myself, but also the planet. Dismissive of those who ate meat, I exuded the self-righteous smugness of one who knows she is right, little realising that such intractability was the result of the copper and zinc imbalance that is a consequence of the diet. Meanwhile, the campaign against red meat and saturated fats was kicking off, and the idea that they were the cause of chronic disease was accepted without question.

I have therefore learnt the hard way that meat and animal fat are an essential part of the human diet. I have also discovered that, far from occupying the moral high ground when it came to the environment, the ecological arguments put forward in support of vegetarianism did not stack up either. There are many myths around vegetarianism which 30 years ago persuaded me that it represented a moral and healthy imperative. Unfortunately, those arguments have subsequently turned out to be specious.

Because of the body's incredible ability to adapt to conditions that are less than ideal, the links between health problems and vegetarianism are not immediately obvious. The body will work hard to keep the metabolic show on the road, but the effects of having to compensate for a diet that is imbalanced, insufficient and toxic will eventually take its toll. Indeed, it is often after a challenge such as pregnancy, illness or stress that the inadequacies of the vegetarian diet start to surface, but these are invariably attributed to the event itself.

So, like a submarine dipping below the radar, vegetarianism can continue its silent erosion of health over many years. Adapting to a steady influx of anti-nutrients without making too much fuss and able to live off stored B12, you are unlikely to notice that your vitality is slowing ebbing away whilst your waistline expands. In spite of the irrefutable case against vegetarianism, so pervasive is the anti-meat/anti-fat lobby that the vegetarian diet is still perceived by many as a healthy way of eating. Indeed, it is sometimes adopted in an attempt to conquer a life-threatening disease.

Vegetarian diets were first introduced to the Western world by the naturopathic heilpraktikers (naturopaths) of Germany and the hapless doctors trying to abate the tide of digestive problems during the Industrial Revolution, little realising the indigestibility of processed grains to have been the cause. Doctors have never been noted for their expertise in nutrition so the connection between diet and indigestion – and, indeed, poor health – evaded them as it does many of their co-professionals today, so various characters attempting to cure indigestion stepped up to fill this gap. Amazingly, no one made the connection with the sudden change in diet (and many still haven't), but since the digestive system comes into direct content with what we eat, it would seem an obvious place to look.

Instead, vegetarianism was proffered as a healthy lifestyle choice and was thus forced down the throats of the previously meat-eating population. They say timing is everything, and with the lack of availability of fresh meat, vegetarianism appealed to many people, not least the food producers who saw an opportunity to feed a growing urban population on mass-produced cheap food with a prolonged shelf life. Transporting meat to cities would have been almost impossible without refrigeration and the combustion engine, evidence perhaps that we should not be living in cities but should be more closely connected to the source of our food.

At his sanatorium in Michigan, Dr John Harvey Kellogg recommended abstinence from meat and developed new 'foods' such as processed soy, peanut butter and breakfast cereals, which you will recognise as a mish-mash of anti-nutrients, indigestible starches and harmful fats. And so the high-sugar breakfast cereal was born. It is ironic that Dr Kellogg's views carried such weight because he himself suffered from obesity, which is not in the least surprising since adopting a vegetarian diet is one of the most efficient methods of fattening up, especially around the middle. Undeterred, however, Dr Kellogg published many articles on health *that still inform our beliefs on diet today, despite the fact that they have no scientific basis.*

The food pyramid (see page 9) touts the wholegrain, high-fibre mantra, with minimal amounts of meat and even less fat. This crazy concept is based on the opinions – yes, 'opinions' – of the aforementioned Dr Kellogg and a Dr Lulu Hunt,[1] who first put forward the idea of calorific restriction for weight loss which has also been shown to be unfounded. This hasn't stopped it being enshrined in medical dogma, which informs dietary thinking today.

You may recall that our original habitat was the African savannah.[2] The savannah differs from the tree-dense environment of primates who eat more vegetation in their diets. Herbivores live off the grasses of the savannah, and omnivores (humans) live off the herbivores rather than directly off the grasses. Moreover, it was only the consumption of animal fat and, in particular, a special fat from the omega-3 family called DHA which is found in bone marrow, that enabled the human brain to increase in size,[3] and the rest, as they say, is history.

## Lose your veg-inity!

Recent research has shown many vegetarian beliefs to have been false, proving unequivocally that humans have more in common with carnivores. In fact, the vegetarian diet, consisting predominantly of foods that were unknown to our Paleo ancestors, actually represents a total reversal of the Stone Age diet. High in carbohydrate from grains and legumes, in polyunsaturated oils and sometimes dairy produce, it can be challenging even to the healthiest physiology.

Relying exclusively upon nutritionally disappointing foods like grains and legumes for protein is unwise because of their relatively low nutritional content and the presence of enzyme inhibitors and phytic acid. Legumes do not provide the full range of amino acids as they lack lysine and methionine but are high in carbohydrates which can be difficult to digest. Although sprouting and fermenting can mitigate their effects and increase their nutritive value, legumes are nutritionally inferior to meat. For this reason, I would not recommend eating them cooked, and would supplement them with other sources of protein, such as meat or fish, if eaten raw as sprouts. In their fermented form they are generally an accompaniment rather than the centrepiece of a meal.

The extensive processing necessary to make them edible, combined with a profusion of anti-nutrients, means the vegetarian diet is, at best, inadequate if not dangerous. The high quantities of carbohydrates that have to be got through in order to obtain protein can encourage weight gain and deplete the digestive system – since the pancreas is ill-equipped to supply enough starch-splitting enzymes, reserves have to be drafted in, leaving the rest of the body undersupplied. The 'dysbiotic' gut of the vegetarian, with standing-room-only for fermenting bacteria, as all resources are directed towards carbohydrate digestion, would displace the good guys needed for immunity – the 'friendly' intestinal bacteria.

Nevertheless, the reason it can take many years for the shortfalls of the vegetarian diet to manifest is because the body will 'adapt'. It is designed to work around problems even if it means robbing Peter to pay Paul. Prioritising resources and drawing on reserves, a gradual and imperceptible decline in health advances as the vegetarian time-bomb ticks silently away. The high demands on the digestive system combined with imbalanced and inadequate levels of nutrients put the body under chronic stress, which is further worsened by the incessant adrenal stimulation of a diet high in sugars. It is only when the body finally runs out of adaptive capacity and becomes exhausted that health problems strike.

According to Hans Seyle's 'general adaptation syndrome' (as described earlier, on page 45), failure to adapt is the third and final phase of stress following the **alarm** and **resistance** stages. Known as the **exhaustion** phase, it manifests when the stressors on the body have exceeded its ability to adapt. Invariably attributed to other factors such as ageing, stress or overwork, exhaustion is frequently marked by the onset of disease. Leaving aside the ethical, religious and cultural aspects of eating animals for the moment, let us have a closer look at why humans are not designed to be vegetarian.

We have hopefully established that the optimal diet for humans is one that is high in saturated fat and low in carbohydrate, and that carbohydrates are not essential unless you are engaged in strenuous exercise, as the body can make them from fat and protein. Given the poor availability of protein from grains and legumes and the denatured state of those found in pasteurised milk, it is evident that the vegetarian diet would struggle to provide enough protein. Furthermore, the unhealthy quantities of carbohydrate that would have to be chomped through would drain the body's vitamin and mineral reserves. I have already discussed the reasons why grains are not healthy, but it may be worth reminding ourselves that until the Industrial Revolution grains were largely used to feed animals, and were supplemental rather than fundamental to the diet.

The hunter-gatherer tradition goes back millions of years. Man belongs to the species Primata, which is thought to have evolved from insect-eating mammals.[4] More than 95 per cent of primates have the single-chambered stomach of the omnivore and carnivore which is not equipped to digest complex carbohydrates, such as those found in grains and legumes, and this is why many people suffer from wind and bloating after eating them. The earliest human remains show that, unlike primates that live in forests and eat a diet higher in vegetation, early humans lived on open plains which they shared with herbivores.

## The high-volume low-return diet

There was a sudden decline in health and stature when we started eating grains. *Homo erectus* of 30,000 years ago was some 150 millimetres (6 inches) taller than his descendants, and we are even shorter today in comparison. There has never been any evidence that humans were herbivorous, and fossil remains consistently show that we have always eaten meat.

## Vegging on the ridiculous

Since the nutrients found in grains are mostly destroyed by milling, eating a predominantly grain-based diet would obviously put you in a state of **negative nutrition** as the vegetarian diet is reliant upon stored nutrients to process it. All carbohydrates are eventually broken down into sugar, but those from vegetables and the less sweet fruits do not raise the blood sugar or stress the pancreas in the way that grains and legumes do. Since unused sugar is stored as fat, grains are excellent for fattening up farm animals, but are best kept to a minimum by everyone else.

Grains may also increase the risk of cancer. One researcher, Stanislaw Tanchou, was able accurately to predict cancer rates based upon the amount of grain consumed in major European cities, showing that the higher the intake, the greater the risk.[5] However, this research needs to be qualified. As the grains consumed today are usually refined and are not adequately prepared by soaking, fermenting or sprouting, the detrimental effects on health would almost certainly have been mediated had they been eaten in a healthier form.

## Fat fantasies

The most damning research as far as vegetarian diets are concerned was carried out in 1972 when it was discovered that about half the human brain and nervous system is made of fats, *but that none of these fats are found in plants*. Plants contain simpler fats which need to be transformed into long chains by animals, and this is where herbivores fit in. Our brain is bigger than that of the ape and about 50 per cent larger than that of cows. The dramatic increase in brain size from ape to man required large quantities of the right fats, particularly DHA, and could never have occurred had our ancestors been vegetarian. Human milk is chock full of these fats whereas cow's milk isn't, and vegetarian staples like soy, nuts and grains lack the saturated fats essential for proper brain development. Although they could be obtained from coconut fat it is the PUFAs that tend to dominate the vegetarian diet. Lacto-ovo vegetarians could obtain cholesterol from dairy produce and eggs, but the vegan would have to make it in the liver. Bone marrow is very rich in fat and it also contains glycoproteins (sugar bound to protein), such as glucosamine and chondroitin, which are good for muscle and joint health but which also cannot be obtained from plant sources.

Those who live nearer the Equator have retained the ability to make EPA and DHA – two fats which are found predominantly in animal foods – out of other omega-3 fats, such as linseeds. Unfortunately, those who live in colder climates are unable to do this conversion since the traditional diet has always been abundant in animal fats. It is true these fats are found in algae, but in lower amounts, and are concentrated by the fish who eat them, making fish a superior source for humans. What's more, the oils in fish are not damaged by cooking unless this is done at a very high temperature, such as deep-fat frying.

As polyunsaturated fats, DHA and EPA are susceptible to rancidity if cooked. It is therefore preferable to eat cured or cold smoked fish or to add raw eggs to smoothies.

## Vitamin B12

Vitamin B12 is an important vitamin necessary for:
- Detoxification
- Nervous system function
- Digestive system function
- Protein metabolism
- To make nucleic acids, which are the building blocks for repair and regrowth
- To make the myelin sheath that protects nerves
- Healthy cell division.

Without B12, incomplete breakdown of a protein called methionine can result in inadequate **homocysteine** metabolism, and this is linked to high blood pressure and Alzheimer's disease.[6]

The mechanisms governing B12 absorption are incompletely understood. However, what is known is that it is a complex process relying upon healthy levels of stomach acid (which is stimulated by animal protein), and pancreatic secretions, a neutral pH in the small intestine (dependent upon the chime leaving the stomach being sufficiently acidic) and healthy biosis. High in carbs, the vegetarian diet is more likely to encourage the overgrowth of starch splitting, fermenting bacteria, and would not stimulate adequate acidity of the stomach. Bacteria are obviously important for B12 uptake, and appear to have a role in releasing it from binding proteins and attaching it to others. An increase in B12 uptake by inhibition of gut bacteria by antibiotics has been recorded, and furthermore unhealthy bacteria compete for dietary B12.[7]

It is well documented that humans are not able to absorb B12 from plants, where it is found in the 'analogue', or copy, form, which can displace the original substance. An analogue is identical to the original but reversed, which is a bit like having the patterns on a key the opposite way round. This is why grasses like green barley and spirulina, although high in B12, can block uptake of this vitamin, and studies on green grasses have indicated that drinking them regularly can lead to deficiency. A vegan diet would fail to provide useable B12 whilst promoting a digestive milieu that would be unfavourable to its absorption. This is why vegans, unless supplementing with B12 *from animal sources* all eventually develop pernicious anaemia. This provides irrefutable evidence that humans are not designed to be vegetarian.[8]

Even if they are fermented or sprouted, grains and legumes have a suppressive effect on stomach acid production because of their high-carb and low-protein content. A vegetarian diet may increase the risk of pernicious anaemia, or B12 deficiency, due to lack of something called 'intrinsic factor', which can only be produced by a stomach with a low pH and why blood levels of B12 drop when antacids are taken.[9]

You may have heard that grasses like green barley and spirulina are high in B12. Unfortunately, the form of B12 they contain is an 'analogue', or copy, of B12, which can block uptake of this vitamin. Studies have shown that green grasses do not raise B12 levels, and in fact drinking them regularly can lead to deficiency. It has been argued that since they show no sign of deficiency, vegetarian Hindus must be able to obtain B12 from plant sources. However, it turns out that they are getting their B12 from insects indigenous to the plants they eat. This is supported by the fact that they become B12 deficient when they move to countries like the UK,[10] where plant foods are likely to have been sprayed with pesticides or scrubbed clean of insects. Incidentally, the vegetarians of southern India tend to have the shortest lifespans in the world.[11] The best source of B12 is organ meats, which are not so popular today, lean muscle meat having generally replaced offal in the modern diet.

## Veggie vitamins

Dr Weston Price discovered that native diets were up to ten times higher than ours in the fat soluble vitamins A, D, E and K. This was due to the large amounts of fat they consumed. Although vitamin D can be absorbed from sunlight, conversion to its active form is dependent upon an adequate supply of cholesterol and efficient liver and kidney function. In more temperate climates such as northern Europe and Scandinavia where sunlight may be in short supply, dietary sources become crucial.

Likewise, beta carotene, the form of vitamin A found in plants, needs to be converted to retinol and not everybody is good at doing this. In those who do manage the conversion it takes 46 units of carotene to make one of retinol.[12] Vitamin A from animal sources like butter comes in the retinol form since the animals do the conversion for us in their intestines. Retinol is necessary for:

- Vision
- Immune function
- Protein metabolism
- Mineral utilisation
- Protection against cancer.

The fat-soluble vitamins are inactive unless accompanied by fat and fat cannot get into the body without bile. Babies and those with hypothyroidism, diabetes or gall bladder problems tend to have a low output of bile. Bile is important because it acts like an emulsifier, making fats digestible and absorbable, in the same way that washing-up liquid pulls grease off pans.

Although grains contain few B vitamins, those they do have are destroyed by milling whilst two vitamins needed to process grains are completely absent. These are the B vitamin biotin, and vitamin C, both of which are needed for immunity, blood sugar regulation, brain function and energy production.

## The iron irony

Iron comes in two forms – 'haem' iron from meat and non-haem iron from plants, eggs and dairy – and there are no prizes for guessing which one we absorb better. Meat contains 40 per cent haem iron and 60 per cent non-haem iron, with an average combined absorption rate of between 20 and 35 per cent. Non-haem iron from plants, however, is bound to phytic acid, which causes the absorption rate to drop to between 2 and 20 per cent. Milk not only contains very little iron but interferes with the assimilation of iron from any other foods eaten at the same meal. Vitamin C, on the other hand, improves iron absorption so eating vegetables with meat is a good idea.

Iron is also needed for energy production and this is why low levels of iron cause tiredness and fatigue. More than two-thirds of the body's iron is found in haemoglobin (the oxygen-carrying red pigment in red blood cells), with smaller amounts in muscles and enzymes. Around 15 per cent of iron is stored in case of a future shortfall in the diet. Whilst vegetarians are found to have normal *circulating* levels of iron, their stored iron is usually found to be low, suggesting that the dietary intake is just about adequate and they are drawing on their reserves.

## The eggs-factor

The iron in eggs is completely bound up by something called a phosphoprotein (phosvitin) otherwise known as the 'egg factor', making it completely useless. It is estimated that one boiled egg will reduce the availability of iron from other foods eaten at the same meal by 28 per cent. This means that vegetarians cannot rely on eggs to meet their iron needs and are going to struggle to extract it from grains and legumes because of the phytic acid problem. Furthermore, foods such as spinach, kale, beetroots, nuts, chocolate, tea, wheat bran, rhubarb, strawberries, oregano, basil and parsley are all high in another acid, oxalic acid, which blocks the uptake of non-haem iron. So Popeye was wrong after all!

## Veggie kids

Most children today are deficient in iron as they only absorb an average of 10 per cent of dietary iron, and rapid growth increases their need for all nutrients, especially iron and zinc.

The iron in breast milk is three times more absorbable compared with formula. In fact, consumption of cow's milk is the most common cause of iron-deficiency anaemia in children as it interferes with iron uptake from other foods whilst providing virtually no iron itself. Cow's milk can also cause intestinal bleeding due to its tendency to irritate the lining of the gut, which would further increase the need for iron. So great is the problem of iron-deficiency anaemia that it is the leading nutritional deficiency in the United States. Formula milks and breakfast cereals are now fortified with it and the American National Institutes of Health recommend all children between the ages of nine and 24 months be regularly screened for anaemia.[13] Iron deficiency in children can delay motor and mental development, causing clumsiness, and also interferes with thinking and processing skills. In teenagers it can affect memory, and in all age groups it causes fatigue as it also helps muscles store and use oxygen.

**Table 5:** Recommended daily intakes for iron in milligrams (mg) depending on age and gender. (Figures from the National Institutes of Health, US)

| Age/Group | Life stage | Iron (mg/day) |
|---|---|---|
| Infants | 0 – 6 months | 0.27, although not enough information is available to be certain |
| | 7 – 12 months | 11 |
| Children | 1 – 3 years | 7 |
| | 4 – 8 years | 10 |
| Males | 9 – 13 years | 8 |
| | 14 – 18 years | 11 |
| | 19 – 30 years | 8 |
| | 31 – 50 years | 8 |
| | 51 – 70 years | 8 |
| Females | 9 – 13 years | 8 |
| | 14 – 18 years | 15 (increased need due to menstruation) |
| | 19 – 30 years | 18 |
| | 31 – 50 years | 18 |
| | 51 – 70 years | 8 |
| | 70+ years | 8 |
| Pregnant women | 14 – 18 years | 27 |
| | 19 – 30 years | 27 |
| | 31 – 50 years | 27 |
| Lactating women | 14 – 18 years | 10 |
| | 19 – 30 years | 9 |
| | 31 – 50 years | 9 |

Brain damage has been found in children on extreme macrobiotic diets, and vegetarian children tend to have growth deficits compared with their meat-eating counterparts. Vegetarian children have only 70 per cent of the energy and 40 per cent of the calcium intake of non-vegetarian children.[14] They also tend to perform less well academically, with 33 per cent failing to complete IQ tests due to poor concentration,[15] although this may be due in part to low levels of animal fats and zinc needed for the brain.

Since children have smaller stomachs than adults it would be impossible for them to obtain adequate nutrition from a plant-based diet. Infertility, miscarriage and increased premature deliveries are associated with vegetarianism together with lower birth weights and smaller head circumference in the offspring – all of which are linked to zinc deficiency.[16] The best source of zinc is oysters and this is why they have a reputation for being aphrodisiac, although good levels can also be found in sea foods and grass-fed meat.

## Disease, longevity and vegetarianism

The mortality rate amongst vegetarians tends to be higher compared to meat eaters, with vegetarian women fairing significantly worse than men. Dr Mercola cites a study carried out by Russell Smith PhD, on heart disease, which demonstrated a decrease in mortality rate which correlated with an increase in the consumption of animal foods. Vegetarians have been shown to have a higher death rate generally, although a slightly reduced incidence of cardiovascular disease.[17] Furthermore, explorers such as Weston Price and Stefansson noted longevity amongst hunter-gatherers such as the Inuit, Polynesians and Australian Aboriginals, all of whom ate a predominantly animal-based diet and whose health deteriorated upon the adoption of the higher carbohydrate diet of 'civilisation'.

Vegetarians have been found to be more at risk from tuberculosis. Those who emigrate from hotter to colder climates but continue to eat their native diet eventually develop vitamin D deficiency. This may be a contributory factor to the increased risk of TB amongst Asians since vitamin D is protective against infections and helps boost immunity. Dark-skinned people from warmer climates are inefficient convertors of vitamin D compared with pale freckly Celts whose bodies are used to making the most of any sunlight they can get.

## You can survive but you won't thrive on a vegetarian diet

There is little doubt today that the vegetarian diet places a strain on the body. Some people, but not me, believe that a vegetarian diet can be therapeutic in the short term – for example, when undertaking detoxification regimes, and this is a hangover from the Kellogg/spa tradition. Since proteins are required to work the detox pathways in the liver, attempting detoxification whilst fasting or trying to survive on fruits and veg is madness, and the thumping headache that is welcomed as a healing crisis is more likely to be due to hypoglycaemia and depletion of a key amino acid needed for detox, glutathione.

Most commonly eaten vegetarian foods, such as refined vegetable oils, soy, unfermented grains and pasteurised dairy products, have only entered the human diet over the last few decades, which suggests the vegetarian diet poses a significant challenge to our hunter-gatherer physiology. Vegetarian meat substitutes are highly processed foods, often derived from soy, and also tend to be loaded with hydrogenated fats ('trans-fats'). Today in the UK and US up to 90 per cent of vegetarian cheese sold in supermarkets has been made from GM rennet derived from soy. This is cheaper than using rennet from cows. Cow genes are inserted into microbes, generally *Aspergillis niger*, to stimulate the production of chymosin, but this produces only one of many possible chymosins. *Aspergillus niger* is commonly found in the guts of children with autism. It is not necessary to label the cheese as GM-derived as soy would be classified as a 'processing agent' and not an ingredient. .

## Copper-bottomed reason for not being veggie

A major problem with vegetarianism is that it raises levels of bio-unavailable copper whilst depleting the body of zinc. This is unfortunate since zinc, along with other minerals, is needed for the metabolism of copper. Copper is an essential mineral but since it binds heavy metals like mercury it could potentially encourage storage rather than elimination of environmental toxins. Copper is also necessary for incorporating calcium into bones and for immunity. When the copper to zinc ratio goes up, copper undergoes a metamorphosis, turning from an essential mineral into a toxin. This I believe is partly responsible for the epidemic of mental illness today, including eating disorders and autism. Copper also raises oestrogen levels and is implicated in hormonal disruption, menstrual problems, reduced sperm counts in males and diseases associated with elevated levels of oestrogen, such as endometriosis, and prostate and breast cancer.

Ironically, one of the first signs that copper is getting out of control is the desire to go vegetarian, probably because of an inability to make enough stomach acid due to declining levels of zinc and vitamin B6. When stomach acid is low meat becomes repugnant and difficult to digest. Low zinc also upsets appetite regulation and is linked to anorexia. Copper can cause feelings of spaciness and idealism which often delude the vegetarian into thinking s/he is having a more spiritual or religious experience due to the lack of flesh in the diet. Unfortunately, high copper also induces intransigence and closed mindedness and this can make it almost impossible to persuade the high-copper/zinc-deficient vegetarian teenager to eat meat.

Vegetarianism often strikes at puberty due to the increased demand for zinc to make hormones which, unless corrected, can eventually lead to the development of mental health problems, including eating disorders. The discovery that animal fats are necessary for the brain and that we require B12 from meat has put the final nail in the vegetarian coffin. Let's now look at whether a vegetarian diet can be a sustainable way of feeding the world.

## The ecological, ethical and environmental implications of vegetarianism

On the face of it, vegetarianism would seem to occupy the higher moral ground but a deeper examination of the issues reveals the arguments to be more complicated. During my zealous vegetarian days I believed that not only human health but planetary health would benefit from vegetarianism, having been persuaded that land used for grazing could be more productively used for the cultivation of grain. However, this argument fails to take into account the fact that only 11 per cent of the earth's surface is suited to arable farming whilst animals can graze on poor quality land – from freezing mountains to sun-baked deserts.

Morally, it is almost impossible to draw a line free of contradictions in support of vegetarianism. Unless going to the extremes of Jainist monks who sweep the ground before them for fear of treading on an insect, the vegetarian could find himself on shaky philosophical ground. Organic vegetarian foods are fertilised with animal manure whilst the non-organic are sprayed with herbicides to kill pests. Male calves and chicks are often culled to concentrate resources on the animals that can produce milk and eggs. Should the vegetarian not wear leather shoes and avoid woollens in the winter? Should she shun cosmetics, toiletries, cleaning products and medicines either because they contain animal products or have been tested on animals? Should she inflict a vegetarian diet on her carnivorous pets? Vegans, who eschew dairy produce and honey, fare little better in the morality stakes as they have to deal with the fact that they will eventually require B12 from animals to save their lives.

Hugh Fearnley-Whittingstall discusses the contradictions and consequences of vegetarianism in his excellent book *The River Cottage Meat Book*,[18] and I share his views. In the book he highlights some of the anomalies in the case for vegetarianism.

Over the centuries animals reared for meat have become domesticated and it would not be easy to return them to the wild, where they would be ill prepared to fend for themselves. Furthermore, whether they would live at all and who would provide land for them would have to be carefully thought through, since land is largely privately owned. If a landowner were magnanimous enough to provide grazing for wild animals, would he then become responsible for their welfare? If not, would he allow them to get old, ill and suffer a lingering death? Would he be obliged to protect them from predators, and in so doing be interfering with the natural order of things by favouring one species over another? In allowing animals to live on his land he would be indirectly rather than directly controlling their deaths. Leaving animals to freeze to death in the winter or to die slowly due to lack of veterinary intervention would seem crueller than a quick death at an abattoir.

As Fearnley-Whittingstall points out, animals are not immortal and so death is inevitable. Would it not be kinder to provide good living conditions throughout their lives, after which they can be humanely killed, rather than leaving them to a slow death from injury, starvation, disease or from being preyed upon by another animal? Moreover, what would happen to these animals after death? Should they be left to decompose, or composted to make fertiliser, and if so, would we not then be eating them indirectly anyway?

In addition, an arable agricultural system would create intense environmental pressures, and would not produce enough to feed everybody. Organic farming is dependent upon animal manures and the integration of both plant and livestock production. As I have said already, vegetarians eating organic produce are eating crops grown from animal manure. The biodiversity of the countryside would be amongst the first casualties in a vegetarian world, resulting in the loss of hedgerows and the demineralisation of the soil, necessitating the use of fertilisers and pesticides, which would in turn make it almost impossible to grow anything organically.

The natural order has always been that herbivores concentrate the nutrients from plants for omnivores and carnivores, who are unable to digest large amounts of vegetation. Nature is not wasteful and every living creature seems to have a part to play. From the big fish that eat the little fish to the carnivores that eat the herbivores, the inter-dependency of one species upon another appears to be a sustainable and viable system with each of us being part of a larger food chain.

Urban life has separated us from the production of our food and we no longer see life as a series of cycles of which death is an integral and essential part. Said by some to be the last taboo, death is often regarded with fear and dread rather than the natural way of balancing regeneration and destruction, of the old making way for the new. Repudiation of death has only become possible since we cocooned ourselves in suburbia. This is probably why vegetarianism first appeared following the Industrial Revolution, when sentimentality rather than rationality started to colour our thinking.

## Mixed and 'mono' farming

Vegetarianism has indirectly contributed to the polarisation of farming today, with the modern trend towards monoculture which is an extremely inefficient way of producing food. On the mixed farms of the past, animals, crops and the land enjoyed a mutually beneficial relationship, with pests being controlled by animals rather than chemicals. According to Mark Purdey,[19] author of *Animal Pharma*, a properly managed mixed farm will yield up to five harvests a year in contrast with the one or two of a mono-cropped farm. A mixed farm is also healthier for the soil, which is replenished by animal waste and crops are rotated, enabling the soil to remineralise. The urine of grazing animals is high in water and nitrogen, which also nourishes the soil, whereas large amounts of water are required for intensively reared animals for both drinking purposes and to clear away waste.

Modern crops, forced by pesticides to grow in demineralised soil, can be up to 80 per cent lower in minerals compared with those grown 50 years ago. Therefore a mixed farm producing livestock and plant foods would be more ecologically tenable and twice as productive than a monofarm producing only plant foods. Moreover, intensive farming in which animals are fed unnatural foods, like soy beans and corn, are indeed wasteful of resources because the crops themselves have first to be cultivated.

## Factory farming

It is difficult to argue against vegetarianism when animals for meat are reared in conditions that no civilised society should tolerate. On the modern battery farm animals subsist in abject misery, frequently ill and in pain and denied access to fresh air and grass. So cramped may be their stalls, they are often unable to turn around or lie down. Furthermore, with its anti-ozone slurry systems, drugs and chemical overuse which have led to diseases such as BSE and CJD, the modern battery farm is wasteful of resources and polluting of the environment. Fed an unnatural diet which may even include animal produce, the quality and nutritional content of factory-farmed meat bear no comparison to those from animals that have been naturally reared. Unsurprisingly, intensively reared animals are highly stressed and may even be lying in their own excrement and in this situation drugs become necessary to control disease.

A staggering 80 per cent of the world's antibiotics are given to farm animals, and indirectly to the humans who eat their meat. Considering how frequently they are prescribed by doctors, this is a truly shocking figure. In 2009 in the USA, the amount of antibiotics given to farm animals weighed in at 13,000 tons and is rising annually. Meat has traditionally been the best source of dietary zinc, but antibiotic-ridden animals become high in copper and low in zinc. The repercussions of this on human health cannot be overstated.

### Slaughter

Hugh Fearnley-Whittingstall is at pains to emphasise our responsibility towards the animals we eat. Animal welfare should be paramount, not only during their lives but at slaughter as well. Whilst people pay lip service to the condemnation of factory farms this does not usually translate to their buying habits, since about 70 per cent of meat sold in the UK is bought from supermarkets.[20] In the UK, around a third of all meat is from animals who were not stunned prior to slaughter. Ten per cent of sheep and goats are not stunned and I have been informed by butchers that one well-known supermarket in the UK sells only un-stunned meat. This issue is raising concern amongst the veterinary profession who claim lack of stunning causes trauma and pain. EU regulations exempt certain religious groups from pre-stunning their animals, but since only 4 to 5 per cent of the population in Britain is Muslim or Jewish, a significant proportion of un-stunned meat is being unknowingly consumed by supermarket shoppers. Non-stun slaughter of sheep and goats increased by 70 per cent between 2003 and 2011 to 1.5 million animals per year according to Peter Harlech-Jones,

President of the British Veterinary Association, which regards this as an animal welfare rather than a religious issue.

For environmental and ethical reasons, it is important that meat eaters take responsibility for how their meat is produced. Buying from a local butcher and questioning him about how and where the meat was reared is essential. Fearnley-Whittingstall witnessed the slaughter of his own animals and was reassured that the process was as painless and stress-free as possible and preferable to most deaths in the wild. This does not mean, however, that all slaughterhouses are as humane as the one he visited. It is important that high standards of animal welfare are rigorously applied. In the UK regulations are more stringent than in many other countries, so cheaper factory farmed meat from abroad sometimes undercuts meat produced in Britain.

However, the transportation of live animals over many miles without food or drink prior to slaughter extends beyond that of animal welfare and becomes an environmental issue as well. Today few slaughtermen are licensed to kill on the farm, but a return to this practice would negate the need for stressful transportation to centralised abattoirs, which themselves are polluting and wasteful of resources. Some of the meat could then be sold through farm shops and local butchers, which would help to ensure the survival of small holdings that currently are under threat from the multi-nationals.

Supermarkets, with their free parking, convenience and ability to slash prices by bulk buying, have largely achieved our co-dependence so it is up to us to exert control over how our food is produced. If enough of us voted with our wallets and shunned intensively reared meat, it would no longer be profitable to produce. Free-range meat would have to come down in price, and animals would no longer have to endure the intolerable conditions to which many are subjected today.

Whilst avoiding meat may appear to palliate the conscience, closer scrutiny of the arguments in favour of vegetarianism shows they don't stack up. The ramifications of feeding the population exclusively from arable produce are insufficiently thought through. Furthermore, anthropomorphism abounds in films and books directed at children, inducing a sentimental attitude towards animals from a young age. The decision to become vegetarian, based on a love of animals and very little in the way of facts, is therefore often inevitable in the sensitive, pubescent copper-toxic child. However, once the physiological and psychological consequences of the diet start to bite, it can often be difficult to reintroduce meat, and thus in some the stage may be set for the development of eating disorders and mental health problems.

That most of us will continue to eat animals in the foreseeable future is beyond dispute. How they are treated and the quality of the meat are the real issues and should command the attention of anyone interested in animal welfare, food or health. If animal welfare were to supersede economic considerations, the disgust that some feel towards eating meat would largely be assuaged. Respect for all life does not mean not killing anything. It means showing care and respect towards animals reared for meat and ensuring they are afforded a quick and humane death at the end of their lives. And that is more than most humans can hope for.

# Chapter 10

# The Paleo paradox

Whether food is a central part of your life or something to be grabbed during a pit stop, it helps define who you are. Your relationship with food is an aspect of your relationship with yourself and it can range from being self-nurturing to self-abusing. For most people today shopping, cooking and eating have to be balanced against the demands of work, family and leisure, which invariably means there will be times when organisation and pre-planning are essential if you want to eat healthily.

No diet should become a religion. The way you eat should enrich your life and not be a source of stress or deprivation. Limiting non-Paleo foods to 20 per cent of the diet usually results in more energy and a reduced risk of degenerative disease. This ratio concurs with the 80/20 rule recommended by Dr Cordain. Processed foods are high in concentrated, refined carbohydrates which are low in fibre. One of the problems with them is that the sugars are so concentrated they interfere with appetite regulation, making it impossible for the body to know when it is full. Regulatory mechanisms, like blood sugar, weight and hormones, can go awry as the body shifts into a state of homeostatic imbalance and cravings take hold. High-sugar foods can become addictive, not only because of their stimulatory effect on the pleasure centre but also because the body becomes reliant upon a cheap energy fix as stimulants such as sugar, tea and coffee take the place of wholefoods.

There is no such thing as a one-size-fits-all diet. What you eat is likely to vary depending on your age, circumstances and activity level. Eating Paleo is not a historic re-enactment of what we assume to have been the Stone Age diet. Diversity is important and prevents the body from becoming reactive to foods when eaten too frequently. Although the modern supermarket may appear to be groaning with produce, the ingredients generally come down to the same few foods; reconstituted soy, refined corn, wheat and salt, and sugar in various guises. Diversity is an illusion, manufactured by synthetic chemicals in order to produce different textures and tastes. The challenge facing manufacturers today is how to supply an urban population with cheap foods that have a long shelf-life. Mass production has led to the loss of many species of fruits and vegetables, in contrast to the hunter-gatherer diet which had a more varied selection of foods from which to choose. Modern meats come from animals selectively bred to be leaner and to reach maturity faster, with little regard for nutritional quality. Today, supermarkets supply 90 per cent of all groceries in the UK, and when the recession bit, organic produce was largely replaced by bargain foods. Since 2008 there has been a drop of 25 per cent in the organic market which, according to Guy Watson, owner of the online supplier Riverford Organic, has made farmers wary of committing to the production of organic food. However, there are encouraging signs that the high street seems to be changing, with artisan shops, farmers' markets and specialist outlets supplanting chain stores who are falling victim to the internet.

In Northern Europe and the Central Mediterranean, the discovery of flour in 30,000-year-old pestles and mortars suggests the division between Paleo and non-Paleo may not have been quite so clear. Although fossilised dental plaque and the remains of barley and tubers have also been found from the Paleolithic period, the fact is that the majority of Paleo foods did not include grains, legumes or dairy. The Paleo philosophy, in common with most philosophies, contains a central grain of truth. It is backed by an impressive body of scientific evidence, but it is impossible for us to go back in time. The Paleo diet can only be understood within the context of the modern age. In the same way that a film about a historical event carries the stamp of the time in which it was made, our understanding of the Paleo diet is inevitably coloured by current beliefs about diet and health and dictated by the food system that serves us today. So there is really no such thing as 'going Paleo'. It could only ever be a modern approximation that followed the spirit of the ancestral diet, and should more accurately be described as 'neo-Paleo'.

Failure to realise this may be why the Paleo diet has attracted criticism. A common argument against it is that it is high in protein and low in vitamin C, both of which criticisms are incorrect. Humans lost the ability to synthesise their own vitamin C in the Eocine period between 56 and 33.9 million years ago, making them dependent upon dietary sources. This is thought to have been an evolutionary adaptation to enhance the storage of fat from fructose . Fruits and vegetables are assumed to be high in vitamin C but this is not supported by the evidence. Vitamin C leeches out the moment the fruit is picked and is also destroyed by cooking, so there is a wide variability in vitamin C levels depending upon ripeness at the time of harvesting, age and method of production. This is one reason why many people today are low in this vitamin – Paleo or not. The average vitamin C content of apples is around 7 per cent with 6 in carrots. Although there is none in muscle meat, beef liver contains a staggering 27 per cent. It is likely that organ meats were the richest source of vitamins in the Stone Age diet, and this is supported by Stefansson, the explorer who travelled with the Inuit, relying upon a meat-based diet to satisfy all his nutritional needs.

Perhaps more than anything your genetic heritage should guide your dietary choices. For instance, if your background was Northern European or Scandinavian and your ancestral diet relied upon fat for warmth, you may be more at risk of blood sugar problems if eating too many carbs. Whether you eliminate grains altogether or demote them from dietary staple to occasional foodstuff is obviously a matter of personal choice. However, autoimmune disease, obesity or a chronic health problem may benefit from complete avoidance – at least for a year or two – after which properly sourced and prepared grains may then be tolerated if eaten every few days. The danger when coming off diets is to go on a bender of the previously forbidden food which can land you back where you started.

Likewise, after a period of elimination, unpasteurised dairy from grass-fed animals may be enjoyed on a rotational basis. The nutrient ratios in sheep and goat milks make them more suited to humans compared with cow, although whether you include milk in your diet depends upon whether you consider it an appropriate food for adults. The poor nutritional quality and limited range of foods available to us today may have made raw butter or ghee essential, regardless of its Paleo credentials. Butter contains a fat called butyric acid (as does milk) which encourages the growth of healthy bacteria in the bowel and can also heal leaky gut. For those with allergies or chronic infections, colostrum or undenatured whey may be helpful in restoring immunity, an issue that would not have arisen in Stone Age times.

Certain health problems could make Paleo eating difficult for some people, and it may be necessary to temporarily restrict the diet to more easily metabolised foods, some of which would not be Paleo. For reasons of practicality, nutrition and variety, trying to implement two diets at one time is never advisable. Salicylates in fruits and vegetables and amines in organ meats are often poorly tolerated by those suffering from environmental illnesses including autism and fatigue disorders. Fermentation too would be out of the question as it increases the amine content of food. Irritable bowel syndrome (IBS), which affects 19 per cent of the population in the UK, may make it impossible to digest certain sugars known as polysaccharides which are found in stoned fruits and vegetables. There are many diets with specific objectives, most of which have some merit.

Psychological factors also have to be taken into account. Refined foods, high in sugar and awash with chemicals, may have caused addictive eating patterns. Childhood is a time when nurture and comfort are important and this is a demographic for whom peer pressure is paramount. Children's parties, those orgies of toxicity that precede hyperactivity, exhaustion and temper tantrums, may be difficult for parents and children alike as dietary considerations intrude upon social activities. This can be quite a challenge as alternative foods would have to pass the discerning toddler taste-test. Not only would they have to appear the same but they would have to be surreptitiously produced at the appropriate time. This requires forward planning (hours in the kitchen), military precision and the collusion of the host parent who may or may not be sympathetic, as your child's diet will inevitably imply criticism of her own.

For some a sudden leap from processed food to Paleo may be a leap too far, not least because of the withdrawal symptoms that may ensue. Children subsisting on a diet of junk foods may struggle to digest fibre, which can be as uncomfortable as it is embarrassing. It may therefore be more feasible at first to provide healthier alternatives, such as soaked grains and raw dairy and to supplement with specialised digestive enzymes. A gradual transition to a low-grain or healthier-grain diet may provide the best strategy, or you may prefer to go cold turkey and eliminate grains altogether. There are plenty of recipe books, including my own *The Urban Caveman*, full of grain-free recipes which would show you how to do this. Alternatively, you may prefer a slower approach by reducing the amount of grains in your diet or just cutting out the gluten-containing grains (wheat, rye, some oats and barley) and substituting millet, for example.

Perfectionism and absolutism have no place in the diet world and it is important to remember that even a small step forward is a step in the right direction. There may be a mountain to climb, but it begins with the first step. Before making any changes to your diet, it is important to make sure you know what you want to gain and what is practicable for you.

The current epidemic of chronic disease is largely the legacy of corporate greed and is not caused by faulty genes or the ageing process. It has altered our physiology and increased our need for nutrients. A baby starting out on pasteurised formula which lacks the immune boosting properties of breast milk may be at a digestive and immunological disadvantage. Plastic bottles and microwaving further damage the milk, increasing the risk of allergies and hormonal imbalances. Being weaned on to processed foods may impede calcium metabolism and blood sugar regulation, and concentrated sources of nutrients may have to be supplemented. For all these reasons, digestive support and mineral balancing may be necessary before moving to a more natural diet. This may mean taking a stomach acid supplement and digestive enzymes. Green vegetable juices are an excellent way of obtaining concentrated minerals in the correct ratios.

## The provenance of food

Factory workers preparing ready meals have replaced the kitchen servants of the past. Unfortunately, such foods require packaging and refrigeration and come with an environmental price tag. Pre-packed sandwiches, made weeks earlier on the other side of the world, which are partially frozen and flown thousands of miles to your local supermarket, obviously require preserving. Preservatives are anti-microbials and are similar to antibiotics. This is great if you want to increase the shelf-life of your food, but not so good for the bacteria in your gut.

We need to rediscover our relationship with the land, with which, until the Industrial Revolution, we have always been intimately connected. Plucked from our natural environment and urbanised in towns and cities, we have been disconnected from our traditional diet, from those who produce our food and from a way of life that has sustained us for millions of years. That is not to suggest that we all move into the country, but if we were to build bridges between our towns and the countryside that surrounds them, we could go some way towards healing ourselves and our environment.

Your diet is not just about what you eat. How your food was produced, the welfare of the animal, whether you buy from a local producer or a corporate, are factors that the responsible consumer needs to consider. Even if you can't buy from a farm shop or farmers' market, you could order from a reputable online producer and relegate the supermarket to the secondary rather than primary provider of your food. Allotments are becoming increasingly popular in the UK and it can be very satisfying to eat vegetables you have grown yourself. Whatever you eat, it should ideally be sustainable and environmentally friendly, not because it is better for you but because you would also be safeguarding the future for your children and grandchildren. Were more of us to distance ourselves from the clutches of the processed food industry the cost of healthy eating would go down, our countryside would be protected from urbanisation and the quality of our food would improve. Supermarkets get away with selling processed food because most of us buy it. Our buying choices determine what they stock. Foods that don't sell disappear overnight. Every time you spend money you vote with your wallet.

I am not suggesting that the world should be transformed into some sort of Paleo paradise. Mechanisation undoubtedly improves the efficiency of crop production and relieves farm workers from the back-breaking and tedious work of the past.

This is a far from perfect world, and compromise is the way we Brits have bumped along in the past. Diets can be a bit of a hot potato – or should I say swede – as they are riven with cultural, moral and religious imperatives. Thank goodness there will never be unanimity on what constitutes the best diet! Even if we have only been eating grains, legumes and dairy for the evolutionary blink of an eye, we cannot ignore 10,000 years of arable farming and the domestication of farm animals. The animals and the foods have become interwoven with the fabric of who we are and have played an important role in shaping the countryside and our cultural identity. Ultimately, all any of us can do is live in accordance with our own conscience.

Tax and health penalties for those who make buying choices that do not conform to someone else's idea of health have no place in a free society. Leaving aside the political lobbying by those with the most to gain (or lose), dietary policy in such a world would be manipulated by the corporates and have little to do with health. The fat phobia that abounds is evidence that this is already happening. As I write, the Food Standards Agency in the UK is currently reviewing whether we should be allowed to consume raw dairy products on the grounds of health and safety. Well, that's the official excuse, but the increasing popularity of unpasteurised dairy produce may be threatening the corporate juggernaut. As governments bow to the corporates, science becomes little more than a marketing tool, and overworked politicians who lack the time to do their own research are steered towards voting in legislation that favours the industry. Profits come before people, but only because most people are unaware this is happening. Were this to continue unchallenged, the brave new world of GM, and industrialised food on a scale never imagined, would be its inevitable consequence. It would make the politically correct food pyramid look like a work of genius.

In this book I have examined the issues as I understand them linked to Paleo eating. Motivated by a desire to make healthy eating enjoyable eating, over the last seven years I have been developing the Urban Caveman diet, which substitutes dairy with coconut milk and cream, and grain-based flours with coconut or nut flours. It wouldn't satisfy the Paleo purists, and it could be argued that coconut products – which have to be transported to parts of the world that would not traditionally have consumed them - lay it open to criticism. However, we no longer forage and limit ourselves to locally sourced, seasonally available foods and coconut has many immune-boosting and healthy properties.

We cannot turn back the clock and return to our old way of living and I doubt that any of us would really want that. The challenge is to integrate the best of the modern world and its technological innovations in a sustainable and ecologically supportive way. Eating fewer grains and going organic would help to relieve the pressures on the earth's resources whilst having a positive impact on our own health. Perhaps more important than the quantitative considerations are the qualitative ones, like mental and emotional wellbeing and having a nurturing environment in which to live and work. Reconnecting with the land could be the beginning of a wonderful and fulfilling relationship, cherishing the inner caveman who – although he loves modern living – also has deep within him an innate link with the natural world. Cutting him off from the countryside has emotional and health consequences that may only be appreciated once that connection were re-established.

The Urban Caveman concept came about as an attempt to reconcile the paradox between two apparently contradictory lifestyles. Just as the Paleo diet needed in my view to be adapted to the 21st century, modern living too may benefit from changes that better suit our inner caveman. Temporarily dazzled by the toys in our technological playroom, we have abandoned our roots. However, rather than becoming polarised – with some townies fleeing to the perceived utopia of the countryside whilst others continue to live the corporate dream in high-rise luxury – perhaps we should instead seek integration. Integrating two ways of life that have until now been unable to coexist may be the next challenge facing humanity.

# References

## Introduction

1. Jones D (2011). Dr Peter Dingel on: Increasing your life expectancy: modern medicine's impact on the extension of life. 2 March.
   www.newdawnmagazine.com

## Chapter one

1. Audette R, Gilchrist T (1999) How our place in the food chain determines our diet. In: *Neanderthin* USA: St Martin's Paperbacks. Page 29.
2. Groves, B (2008) Homocarnivorous. In: *Trick and Treat* London: Hammersmith Press. Pages 200-203.

## Chapter two

1. Cordain L (2012) Grains are anti-nutritious. In: *The Paleo Answer*. John Wiley and Sons Inc. New Jersey: Page 113.
2. Cordain L (2012) Grains are anti-nutritious. In: *The Paleo Answer*. New Jersey, USA: John Wiley and Sons Inc. Page 113.
3. Cordain L (2012) Grains are anti-nutricious. In: *The Paleo Answer*. New Jersey, USA: John Wiley and Sons Inc. Page 116.
4. Klinghardt D (2009) London Conference: Roadmap to Recovery. www.theklinghardtacademy.com
5. Brown B. Coeliac disease and gluten sensitivity: is gluten really to blame? *CAM Journal*: Sept 2013. Page 14.

6.    Fallon S. President's Message: Myths and Truths about the
      Weston Price Foundation: Myth: the WAPF diet is like the Paleo
      diet. *Journal - Wise Traditions*: Summer 2013. The Weston Price
      Foundation, USA. Page 2.
7.    Fallon S. *Caustic Commentary: Journal - Wise Traditions*: Summer
      2013: Page 14. Published by The Weston Price Foundation, USA.
8.    Cordain L. (2012) Grains are anti-nutricious. In: *The Paleo Answer*.
      New Jersey, USA: John Wiley and Sons Inc. Page 119.
9.    O'Brien T (2011) Seminar at Nutri-Link on Gluten. www.theDr.
      com
10.   Cordain L (2012) Grains are anti-nutricious. In: *The Paleo Answer*
      New Jersey, USA: John Wiley and Sons Inc. Page 119.
11.   Wilson L (2010) *Nutritional Balancing and Hair Mineral Analysis*
      Arizona, USA: The Center for Development Inc.
12.   Audette R, Gilchrist T (1999) Why agricultural foods are bad for
      you. In: *Neanderthin – Eat like a caveman to achieve a lean, strong,
      healthy body* USA: St Martin's Paperbacks. Page 54.
13.   Groves B (2008) Climb off the bran wagon. In: *Trick or Treat*.
      London: Hammersmith Press. Page 118-128.
14.   Cordain L (2010) Grains are antinutritious. In: *The Paleo Answer*.
      New Jersey, USA: John Wiley and Sons Inc. Pages 118-119.

## Chapter three

1.    Cordain L (2012) Just say no to the milk moustache. In: *The Paleo
      Answer*. New Jersey, USA: John Wiley and Sons Inc. Page 74.
2.    Segall JJ. Plausibility of dietary lactose as a coronoary risk factor.
      *Journal of Nutritional and Environmental Medicine* 2002; 12: 217-229.
3.    Cordain L ( 2012) Just say no to the milk moustache. In: *The Paleo
      Answer*. New Jersey, USA: John Wiley and Sons Inc. Page 83.
4.    Cordain L (2012) Just say no to the milk moustache. In: *The Paleo
      Answer*. New Jersey, USA: John Wiley and Sons Inc. Page 85.
5.    Cordain L (2012) Just say no to the milk moustache. In: *The Paleo
      Answer*. New Jersey, USA: John Wiley and Sons Inc. Page 86.
6.    Cordain L (2012) Just say no to the milk moustache. In: *The Paleo
      Answer*. New Jersey, USA: John Wiley and Sons Inc. Page 89.
7.    Cordain L (2012) Just say no to the milk moustache. In: *The Paleo
      Answer*. New Jersey, USA: John Wiley and Sons Inc. Page 88.

8.  Cordain L (2012) Just say no to the milk moustache. In: *The Paleo Answer*. New Jersey, USA: John Wiley and Sons Inc. Page 95.
9.  Cordain L (2012) Just say no to the milk moustache. In: *The Paleo Answer*. New Jersey, USA: John Wiley and Sons Inc. Page 95.
10. Cordain L (2012) Just say no to the milk moustache. In: *The Paleo Answer*. New Jersey, USA: John Wiley and Sons Inc. Page 95.
11. Cordain L (2012) Just say no to the milk moustache. In: *The Paleo Answer*. New Jersey, USA: John Wiley and Sons Inc. Page 93.
12. Cordain L (2012) Just say no to the milk moustache. In: *The Paleo Answer*. New Jersey, USA: John Wiley and Sons Inc. Page 96.
13. Audette R, Gilchrist T (1999) *Neanderthin – Eat Like a Caveman to Achieve a Lean, Strong, Healthy Body*. USA: St Martin's Paperbacks.
14. Audette R, Gilchrist T (1999) *Neanderthin – Eat Like a Caveman to Achieve a Lean, Strong, Healthy Body*. USA: St Martin's Paperbacks.
15. Audette R, Gilchrist T (1999) *Neanderthin – Eat Like a Caveman to Achieve a Lean, Strong, Healthy Body*. USA: St Martin's Paperbacks. Page 98.
16. Cordain L (2010) Food Allergies and Colic. In: *The Paleo Answer*. New Jersey, USA: John Wiley and Sons Inc. Page 97.
17. Cordain L (2010) Parkinson's Disease. In: *The Paleo Answer*. New Jersey, USA: John Wiley and Sons Inc. Page 100.
18. Simoons FJ. A geographic approach to senile cataracts. Possible links with milk consumption, lactase activity and galactose metabolism. *Digestive Diseases and Science* 1982; 27(3): 257-264.
19. Cordain L (2012) Just say no to the milk moustache. In: *The Paleo Answer*. New Jersey, USA: John Wiley and Sons Inc. Pages 100-101.
20  Ward NI, Watson R, Bryce-Smith D. Placental element levels in relation to fetal development for obstetrically normal births: a study of 37 elements. Evidence for the effects of cadmium, lead and zinc on fetal growth and smoking as a cause of cadmium. *International Journal of Bioscience Research* 1987; 9(1): 63-81.
21. Cohen R (1998) A brief history of milk in America. In: *Milk The Deadly Poison* USA: Argus Publishing. Page 13.
22. Cohen R (1998) A brief history of milk in America. In: *Milk The Deadly Poison*. USA: Argus Publishing. Page 16.
23. Cohen R (1998) A brief history of milk in America. In: *Milk The Deadly Poison* USA: Argus Publishing. Page 17.

24. Cohen R (1998) A brief history of milk in America. In: *Milk The Deadly Poison* USA: Argus Publishing. Pages 22-23.
25. Peskin BS (2007) The 24-Hour-Diet: Fats: Everything Your Haven't Heard But Need To Know Texas, USA: Pinnacle Press. Page 116.
26. www.westonaprice.org/Splendor from the Grass. Posted on Sept 30 2000 by Sally Fallon and Mary G Enig PhD.
27. Cordain L (2012) Just say no to the milk moustache. In: *The Paleo Answer* New Jersey, USA: John Wiley and Sons Inc. Page 103.

## Chapter four

1. Cordain L (2012) The Paleo Answer: The Trouble with Beans. John Wiley and Sons Inc. New Jersey, US. Page 133.
2. Cordain L (2012) Just say no to the milk moustache. In: *The Paleo Answer* New Jersey, USA: John Wiley and Sons Inc. Page 136.
3. Cordain L (2012) Just say no to the milk moustache. In: *The Paleo Answer* New Jersey, USA: John Wiley and Sons Inc. Page 137.
4. Cordain L (2012) Just say no to the milk moustache. In: *The Paleo Answer* New Jersey, USA: John Wiley and Sons Inc. Page 138.
5. Cordain L (2012) Just say no to the milk moustache. In: *The Paleo Answer* New Jersey, USA: John Wiley and Sons Inc. Page 146.
6. Cordain L (2012) Just say no to the milk moustache. In: *The Paleo Answer* New Jersey, USA: John Wiley and Sons Inc. Page 146.
7. Cordain L (2012) Just say no to the milk moustache. In: *The Paleo Answer* New Jersey, USA: John Wiley and Sons Inc. Page 138.
8. Cordain L (2012) Just say no to the milk moustache. In: *The Paleo Answer* New Jersey, USA: John Wiley and Sons Inc. Page 139.
9. Cordain L (2012) Just say no to the milk moustache. In: *The Paleo Answer* New Jersey, USA: John Wiley and Sons Inc. Page 140.
10. Cordain L (2012) Just say no to the milk moustache. In: *The Paleo Answer* New Jersey, USA: John Wiley and Sons Inc. Page 144.
11. Cordain L (2012) Just say no to the milk moustache. In: *The Paleo Answer* New Jersey, USA: John Wiley and Sons Inc. Page 144.
12. Cordain L (2012) Just say no to the milk moustache. In: *The Paleo Answer*. New Jersey, USA: John Wiley and Sons Inc. Page 145.

## Chapter five

1. Groves B (2008) Soy, fluoride and the thyroid. In: *Trick and Treat*

# References

London: Hammersmith Books Limited. Pages 156-166

2.  Mercola JM (2011) Doctor Warns: 'Eat this and you'll look 5 years older' www.articles.mercola.com 'The dirty little secret hidden in much of your health food. 8 Dec.

3.  Mercola JM (2010) The truth about soy foods: can soy damage your health? www.articles.mercola.com: 18 Sept.

4.  Mercola JM (2010) The truth about soy foods: can soy damage your health? www.articles.mercola.com: 18 Sept.

5.  Fallon S (2000) The Tragedy of Soy Infant Formula. www.westonaprice.org/soy-alert/tragedy-of-soy-formula

6.  Mercola JM (2011) Doctor Warns: 'Eat this and you'll look 5 years older' www.articles.mercola.com 'The dirty little secret hidden in much of your health food.

7.  Fallon S (2000) The Tragedy of Soy Infant Formula www.westernaprice.org/soy-alert/tragedy-of-soy-formula

8.  Groves B (2008) Soy, Fluoride and the Thyroid. In: *Trick and Treat*. London: Hammersmith Press. Page 156-166.

9.  Fallon S (2000) The Tragedy of Soy Infant Formula www.westonaprice.org/soy-alert/tragedy-of-soy-formula

10. Fallon S (2000) The Tragedy of Soy Infant Formula www.westonaprice.org/soy-alert/tragedy-of-soy-formula

11. Mercola JM (2011) Doctor Warns: 'Eat this and you'll look 5 years older' www.mercola.com. 8 Dec.

12. Groves B (2008). Soy, Fluoride and the Thyroid. In: *Trick and Treat*. London: Hammersmith Press. Page 163.

13. Fallon S (2000) The Tragedy of Soy Infant Formula www.westonaprice.org/soy-alert/tragedy-of-soy-formula

14. Mercola JM (2011) Doctor Warns: 'Eat this and you'll look 5 years older' www.mercola.com. 8 Dec.

15. Fallon S (2000) The Tragedy of Soy Infant Formula: www.westonaprice.org/soy-alert/tragedy-of-soy-formula

16. Mercola JM (2011) Doctor Warns: 'Eat this and you'll look 5 years older' www.mercola.com. 8 Dec.

17. www.people.csail.mit.edu/seneff.

18. articles.mercola.com/sites/.../glyphosate-roundup-levels

19. Fallon S (2000) The Tragedy of Soy Infant Formula: www.westonaprice.org/soy-alert/tragedy-of-soy-formula

20. Fallon S (2000) The Tragedy of Soy Infant Formula: www.

westonaprice.org/soy-alert/tragedy-of-soy-formula

21. Peat R (2006) raypeat.com/articles/articles/coconut-oil.

22. Peat R (2006) raypeat.com/articles/articles/coconut-oil.

## Chapter six

1. Cordain L (2012) Grains are anti-nutritious. In: *The Paleo Answer* New Jersey, USA: John Wiley and Sons Inc. Page 121.

2. Cordain L (2012) Grains are anti-nutritious. In: *The Paleo Answer* New Jersey, USA: John Wiley and Sons Inc. Page 122.

3. Cordain L (2012) Grains are anti-nutritious. In: *The Paleo Answer* New Jersey, USA: John Wiley and Sons Inc. Page 122.

4. Cordain L (2012) Grains are anti-nutritious. In: *The Paleo Answer* New Jersey, USA: John Wiley and Sons Inc. Page 122.

5. Cordain L (2012) Grains are anti-nutritious. In: *The Paleo Answer* New Jersey, USA: John Wiley and Sons Inc. Pages 123-4.

6. Cordain L (2012) Grains are ant-inutritious. In: *The Paleo Answer* New Jersey, USA: John Wiley and Sons Inc. Page 124.

7. Cordain L (2012) Grains are anti-nutritious. In: *The Paleo Answer* New Jersey, USA: John Wiley and Sons Inc. Page 126.

8. Cordain L (2012) Grains are anti-nutritious. In: *The Paleo Answer* New Jersey, USA: John Wiley and Sons Inc. Page 127.

9. Cordain L (2012) Grains are anti-nutritious. In: *The Paleo Answer* New Jersey, USA: John Wiley and Sons Inc. Page 128.

10. Cordain L (2012) Grains are anti-nutritious. In: *The Paleo Answer* New Jersey, USA: John Wiley and Sons Inc. Page 128.

11. Cordain L (2012) Grains are anti-nutritious. In: *The Paleo Answer* New Jersey, USA: John Wiley and Sons Inc. Page 129.

12. Cordain L (2012) Grains are anti-nutritious. In: *The Paleo Answer* New Jersey, USA: John Wiley and Sons Inc. Page 153.

13. Cordain L (2012) Potatoes should stay underground. In: *The Paleo Answer* New Jersey, USA: John Wiley and Sons Inc. Page 154.

14. Cordain L (2012) Potatoes should stay underground. In: *The Paleo Answer* New Jersey, USA: John Wiley and Sons Inc. Page 155.

15. Cordain L (2012) Potatoes should stay underground. In: *The Paleo Answer* New Jersey, USA: John Wiley and Sons Inc. Page 157.

16. Cordain L (2012) Potatoes should stay underground. In: *The Paleo Answer* New Jersey, USA: John Wiley and Sons Inc. Page 159.

17. Cordain L (2012) Potatoes should stay underground. In: *The Paleo Answer*New Jersey, USA: John Wiley and Sons Inc. Page 160.
18. Cordain L 2012) Potatoes should stay underground. In: *The Paleo Answer* New Jersey, USA: John Wiley and Sons Inc. Page 160.
19. Furmaga-Jablonska W et al. Fried potato chips and French fries – Are they safe to eat? *Nutrition* 2011; 27(**10**): 1076-1077.
20. Cordain L (2012) Potatoes should stay underground. In: *The Paleo Answer* New Jersey, USA: John Wiley and Sons Inc. Page 148-152.

# Chapter seven

1. Enig MG (2000) The Skinny on Fats. www.westonprice.org/ know-your-fats/skinny-on-fats
2. Peat R (2006) raypeat.com/articles/articles/coconut-oil.
3. Peat R (2006) raypeat.com/articles/articles/coconut-oil.
4. Peat R (2006) raypeat.com/articles/articles/coconut-oil.
5. Rose G, Tunstall-Pedoe H, Heller R. The United Kingdom Heart Disease Prevention Project. Incidence and Mortality Rates. *Lancet* 1983; 1: 1062-1065.
6. Castelli, W. Concerning the possibility of a nut... *Archives of Internal Medicine* 1992; 152(7): 1371-1372.
7. Mercola JM (2013) Omega-6 Fats in Processed and Deep Fried Foods Can Massively Increase Your Heart Disease Risk. *Enewsletter: mercola.com* Feb 21.
8. BioLab Conference (2012) From Autism to Alzheimer's. London. www.greatplainslaboratory.com/.../London-Conference-Brochure.pdf
9. Puotinen CJ. Unhealthy Vegetable Oils? Does Food Industry Ignore Science Regarding Polyunsaturated Oils? *Wellbeing Journal* 2006. www.wellbeingjournal.com/understanding-fats-and-oils/
10. Puotinen CJ. Unhealthy Vegetable Oils? Does Food Industry Ignore Science Regarding Polyunsaturated Oils? *Wellbeing Journal* 2006 www.wellbeingjournal.com/understanding-fats-and-oils/
11. Gorbunov, NV. Effect of structural modification of membrane proteins on lipid-protein interactions in the human erythrocyte membrane. *Bulletin of Experimental Biology & Medicine* 1993; 116(11): 1364-1367.
12. Gorbunov, NV. Effect of structural modification of membrane

proteins on lipid-protein interactions in the human erythrocyte membrane. *Bulletin of Experimental Biology & Medicine* 1993; 116(11): 1364-1367.

13. Gorbunov, NV. Effect of structural modification of membrane proteins on lipid-protein interactions in the human erythrocyte membrane. *Bulletin of Experimental Biology & Medicine* 1993; 116(11): 1364-1367.

14. Enig M (2000) The Skinny on Fats www.westonaprice.org/know-your-fats/skinny-on-fats

15. Moon RJ et al. Maternal plasma polyunsaturated fatty acid status in late pregnancy is associated with offspring body composition in childhood. *The Journal of Clinical Endocrinology and Metabolism* 2012; 98(1): 299-307.

16. Wilson N (2013) drnevillewilson.com/tag/sydney-diet-heart-study/ 10 Feb. www.Paleodietnewsletter.Mar2013 Interview with Dr L Cordain commenting on N Wilson's work.

17. Puotinen CJ. Unhealthy Vegetable Oils? Does Food Industry Ignore Science Regarding Polyunsaturated Oils? *Wellbeing Journal* 2006 www.wellbeingjournal.com/understanding-fats-and-oils/

18. Antoniou M: WAPFConf.Ldn2014.

# Chapter eight

1. Mercola JM. Is Sugar More Addictive than Cocaine? www.mercola.com August-06-2007

2. Assilem M (1994) Saccharaum Officinarum – The Sugar Story. In: *The Mad-Hatter's Tea Party*. The Homeopathic Supply Company. Page 41.

3. Assilem M (1994) Saccharaum Officinarum – The Sugar Story'. In: *The Mad-Hatter's Tea Party*. The Homeopathic Supply Company. Page 41.

4. Barton L. A spoonful of propaganda. *Guardian* 12 April 2002.

5. Barton L. A spoonful of propaganda. *Guardian* 12 April 2002.

6. Barton L. A spoonful of propaganda. *Guardian* 12 April 2002.

7. Scot-Peskin B (2007) Carbohydrates: Sugar in Disguise. In: The 24 Hour Diet. [Pinnacle Press, Houston, Texas]: page 60.

8. No Sweet Surrender. *BMJ* 7 April 2005;330:853,2.

9. Lawrence F. Sugar Rush. *Guardian* 13 Feb 2007.
10. Lawrence F. Sugar Rush. *Guardian* 13 Feb 2007.
11. Lawrence F. Sugar Rush. *Guardian* 13 Feb 2007.
12. Lawrence F. Sugar Rush. *Guardian* 13 Feb 2007.
13. Lawrence F. Sugar Rush *Guardian* 13 Feb 2007.
14. Lawrence F. Sugar Rush. *Guardian* 13 Feb 2007.
15. Lawrence F. Sugar Rush. *Guardian* 13 Feb 2007.
16. Lawrence F. Sugar Rush. *Guardian* 13 Feb 2007.
17. Lawrence F. Sugar Rush. *Guardian* 13 Feb 2007.

# Chapter nine

1. Peters, L (1918). *Diet and Health: With Key to the Calories*. Baltimore: Reilly and Lee. ISBN 1-148-38661-0.
2. Peters L (1918) *Diet and Health: With Key to the Calories*. Baltimore: Reilly and Lee.
3. Cordain L (2002) How our diet went wrong and what you can do about it. In: *The Paleo Diet* New Jersey, USA: John Wiley and Sons, Inc. Page 39.
4. Cordain L (2002) How our diet went wrong and what you can do about it. In: *The Paleo Diet* New Jersey, USA: John Wiley and Sons. Pages 29–35.
5. Audette R, Gilchrist T (2000) Neanderthin: How a Stone Age Diet saved my Life. St Martin's Press USA. Page 20.
6. Mercola M (2000) www.articles.mercola.com/The fallacy of vegetarian diets
7. Schjonsby H. Vitamin B12 absorption and malabsorption. *Gut* 1989; 30: 1686-1691.
8. Schjonsby H. Vitamin B12 absorption and malabsorption. *Gut* 1989; 30: 1686-1691.
9. Schjonsby H. Vitamin B12 absorption and malabsorption. *Gut* 1989; 30: 1686-1691.
10. Mercola M (2000) www.articles.mercola.com/The fallacy of vegetarian diets
11. Mercola M (2000) www.articles.mercola.com/The fallacy of vegetarian diets
12. Byrnes Dr Stephen. Paper: The Myths of Vegetarianism. www.westonaprice.org/vegetarianism-and-plant.../myths-of-

vegetarianism

13. Medline Plus (2012) Iron Deficiency Anemia. www.nlm.nih.gov/
    medlineplus/ency/article/007134.htm

14. Medline Plus (2012) Iron Deficiency Anemia. www.nlm.nih.gov/
    medlineplus/ency/article/007134.htm

15. Medline Plus (2012) Iron Deficiency Anemia. www.nlm.nih.gov/
    medlineplus/ency/article/007134.htm

16. Ward NI, Watson R, Bryce-Smith D. Placental element levels in
    relation to fetal development for obstetrically normal births: a
    study of 37 elements. Evidence for the effects of cadmium, lead
    and zinc on fetal growth and smoking as a cause of cadmium.
    *International Journal of Bioscience Research* 1987; 9(1): 63-81.

17. Mercola M (2000) www.articles.mercola.com/The fallacy of
    vegetarian diets

18. Fearnley-Whittingstall H (2004) *The River Cottage Meat Book*
    London, UK: Hodder and Stoughton.

19. Purdey M (2007) *Animal Pharma* East Sussex, UK: Clairview
    Books.

20. Purdey M (2007) *Animal Pharma* East Sussex, UK: Clairview
    Books. Page 49.

# Index

# Index

## Also by Eve Gilmore

# The Urban Caveman

### *Paleo-friendly recipes for the 21st century*

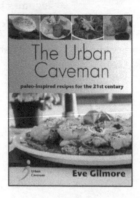

*You can have your cake and eat it!*

In The Urban Caveman, Eve Gilmore brings the Paleo diet into the present day, satisfying our contemporary cravings for comfort foods and complex flavours while maintaining the principles of excluding grains, dairy, sugar and legumes. Different to all other Paleo recipe books, you will find out how to make grain-free, low-carb breads and cakes, creamy desserts and even cheeses, and to replicate favourite foods, like pizza and ice-cream.

With over 300 original recipes, tried and tested by the author and her many clients, with illustrations direct from the author's kitchen, The Urban Caveman shows you how giving up does not mean going without.

**www.hammersmithbooks.co.uk**

**www.21stcenturypaleo.com**